The Covid-19 Crisis

Health and Patients Set

coordinated by
Bruno Salgues

Volume 4

The Covid-19 Crisis

From a Question of an Epidemic to a Societal Questioning

Edited by
Bruno Salgues
Jacques Barnouin

ISTE

WILEY

First published 2022 in Great Britain and the United States by ISTE Ltd and John Wiley & Sons, Inc.

ISTE Ltd
27-37 St George's Road
London SW19 4EU
UK

www.iste.co.uk

John Wiley & Sons, Inc.
111 River Street
Hoboken, NJ 07030
USA

www.wiley.com

Library of Congress Control Number: 2022933262

British Library Cataloguing-in-Publication Data
A CIP record for this book is available from the British Library
ISBN 978-1-78630-726-2

Contents

Introduction

The World after the Coronavirus Pandemic

Observations and facts have taught us that human societies are never ready for change. "[...] the new does not grow out of the old but appears alongside of it and eliminates it competitively" is how Schumpeter described change. The project initiated by this book seeks to reflect on the changes and questions generated by the SARS-CoV-2 pandemic, by analyzing the facts and their consequences on society and institutions, as well as on individual behavior.

The current pandemic can only be the ignitor of the necessary break with the old social, economic and cultural paradigm. It will be a question of describing, guiding and analyzing this break, as well as of contributing to its inevitability, while maintaining it within the framework of the Declaration of the Rights of Man and of the Citizen[1]. To this end, we could take up the intellectual framework defined, deployed and supported by Saint-Simonism in its humanist version. This ideological current had an important influence on the development of industrial society in the 19th century. It thought both of the future and of the individual in that future. This new ignition – post-coronavirus – cannot be unrelated to knowledge, science and the state of the art of technology.

So the global pandemic is here. It is a new threat. However, we are not at the end of *the* world, but at the end of *a* world, hence the importance of

---

Introduction written by Jacques BARNOUIN and Bruno SALGUES.

1 A human civil rights document from the French Revolution.

asking ourselves about the "day after". This is why it is essential to take a forward-looking approach, in which science and technology will take on their full meaning, namely in the service of shared progress and not just the financialization of the innovations they lead to. The Saint-Simonians provided a positive framework for the notion of progress – later taken up by Auguste Comte – in which talent and solidarity, as well as entrepreneurship and general interest, are linked.

However, the view of these political, social and cultural aspirations remained indicative and critical. For half a century, especially during the Second Empire, all Saint-Simonian action was to be systematically devoted to developing "material" networks (communication infrastructures) and "immaterial" networks (institutions of knowledge and credit), which were linked and necessary for the balance between science and society, markets and human communities.

In order to talk about the "day after", multi-author books will have to address the scientific issues linked to information and communication technologies (ICTs) in the major fields of security, health and education and culture, but also analyze the role and actions of these technologies in relation to work and social cohesion. Furthermore, we must not forget the question of the reinvention of democracy in the face of otherness and the need to adapt, under the weight of the influence of technologies with an absolutely manifest power to transform.

Living is an individual risk. Living in a human community is a collective risk.

In this respect, contemporary geopolitical divides have, in recent years, led to the emergence of violence and reality in our domestic spheres, in Europe, but not only so. Therefore, we are witnessing:

– the emergence of a culture of risk and of threat. Threats have indeed started a cycle of psychological changes in the individual;

– an evolution in the way of thinking about our space and intimate domain, through the use of technologies;

– the obligation to look at the political object and its different figures of power through science and knowledge.

These fields inevitably come into contact with the underlying questions of algorithms, heuristic models and artificial intelligence. Above all, they call into question the individual as a citizen with regard to their public liberties and the illusory control of their private data. Here again, the pandemic has raised questions, for health purposes, about the data from applications for tracking movement.

After all crises, new technological and global companies are born. Thus, Watson federated companies in 1914 and proposed the first computer, the Mark I, in 1945. As for Microsoft, the company appeared after the 1973 oil crisis, and the same was true of Uber and WhatsApp in 2009, after the subprime crisis. The list goes on. What companies will emerge as a result of the Covid-19 crisis and, in turn, in which sectors should the biggest research efforts be made?

Finally, the world in disarray will disrupt the notion of territory. On this point, we should not forget the notions of threat and risk, as well as the socio-political context. During the Cold War, the "communist threat" led to the creation of the Coordinating Committee for Multilateral Export Controls (COCOM), a Paris-based organization whose initial goal was to prevent countries under the influence of the Soviet Union or China from importing scientific knowledge and technology. This included goods, materials and technologies of a military nature and of strategic interest, such as transport technology, computers, software and sophisticated telephone exchange equipment. However, COCOM was dissolved on March 31, 1994. Its successor, the Wassenaar Arrangement, was established in 1996 to counter the threat of state terrorism. Are pandemics our new threats?

Historical sequencing is possible between:

– the beginning of the Enlightenment and the rise of industrialization;

– the de-industrialization of the Western world to the benefit of other countries during the 1980s and 1990s, while during this same period, the regalian domains, such as health or education, did not industrialize;

– the situation imaginable after the Covid-19 crisis.

This current and historical sequence is at the origin of refoundations to which we want to contribute, in various scientific and technical fields. These refoundations will not only be enriched by reflections and the putting forward of principles, but also by scientific and sociological creations, the creation of technological tools and state, entrepreneurial and inter-civilizational rules of operation. Basically, the Covid-19 crisis appears to be a sort of avatar of *laissez aller, laisser faire*[2] or *laissez-faire, laisser passer*[3], according to the formula attributed to Vincent de Gournay, who is considered to have introduced economic liberalism to France in the 18th century. Thus, it does not seem conceivable that we will be able to overcome future health crises, whether their origin is microbiological, toxic, linked to unconventional pathogens (let us recall the prion), climatic, economic, political or technological – or multifactorial – without forcing ourselves to fundamentally question ourselves through the implementation of a new social contract shared by nations.

This book brings together the analyses, ideas and proposals of contributors from different backgrounds, including business, academia, research and civic life, who bring experience and expertise from various specialties and life experiences ranging from biology to sociology and technological and organizational sciences. It is therefore a work "written on the spot" that the reader will discover, a work updated at the time of publication, but which, in addition to analyzing the epidemic and its "side effects", aims to lay down milestones, relating experiences and reporting reactions with the idea of proposing and building. As for the writing of the text, itself marked by the diversity of the themes, the statements and the authors, it ranges from the scientific style to that of the academic essay, passing through the style of testimonies, the reporting of experiences and personal reflections.

Our thoughts are with all those who left this world – much too soon – because of the pathogenicity of the SARS-CoV-2 virus, its unfavorable biological and health traits, the unpreparedness of health systems and the lack of scientific knowledge. As for the contributors of this book, they have experienced, like so many, painful and significant losses and difficult separations, whether from parents, loved ones, acquaintances or iconic figures. Losses and separations reveal, on the one hand, dysfunctions (imperfections, unconsciousness, rapacity) and, on the other hand, magnificence (caregivers, helpers, the voices of the lonely). May the Covid-19 crisis, which could have been mastered, prove to be an opportunity to develop new practices, new solidarities, new antivirals, new technologies

2 Literally, this means "letting go, leaving alone".

3 Literally, this means "leaving alone, leaving it to happen".

of care and new tools for epidemic prevention, in which everyone should be an actor, insofar as health is everyone's business. May it be an opportunity to act in order to protect the stakes of public health from commercial competition and economic deregulation, through the implementation of an organized and obligatory cooperation of States around these stakes, cooperation concerning, at the same time, research, production and distribution of molecules and essential materials. All this with the aim of turning the health crisis into an opportunity for the human race.

This book is built around Covid-19. The first finalized texts serve as reflections, complements and elements of controversy for other researchers, and also for actors from the economic and social sphere. New ideas may be added in future texts, thus constituting a body of ideas and proposals for the "day after". The announcements of prolonged states of health emergency in many countries, as we finish this book, suggest that this day after is not for tomorrow.

1

Deciphering the Covid-19 Epidemic and Analysis of Its Controllability

1.1. Facts and lessons learned from the emergence of Covid-19 in France

1.1.1. *SARS-CoV-2 and emerging risks*

The emergence of the severe acute respiratory syndrome coronavirus 2 (SARS-CoV-2) virus (Figure 1.1), which resulted in the appearance in central China in fall 2019 (Wu and McGoogan 2020) of an atypical pneumonia, coronavirus disease 2019 (Covid-19), was followed by its development into a major pandemic. This pandemic, which had a particular impact on France, led to a strong health mobilization throughout the world. Before developing the subject, it is appropriate to pay tribute to the victims of Covid-19, that is, officially, about 6 million people worldwide (between January and September 2020, while 1 million people had already lost their lives as a result of SARS-CoV-2, there were also 320,000 victims of malaria, 340,000 victims of influenza, 780,000 victims of AIDS, 1.2 million deaths linked to road accidents and 3.6 million deaths linked to smoking (Planetoscope 2020)).

Covid-19 disease is the consequence of infection by a virus: emerging (new and with uncertain consequences) from the *Coronaviridae* family; single-stranded RNA (ribonucleic acid), like the influenza virus; highly contagious (one infected person can infect two to four or even eight healthy people, depending on the strain), probably because it settles in the upper

Chapter written by Jacques BARNOUIN.

respiratory tract and is thus easily re-excreted via coughing or sneezing; average incubation time of two to six days (Sanche et al. 2020); highly resistant in the environment (resistant for up to 28 days at 20°C on smooth surfaces, but only 24 h at 40°C) (Riddell et al. 2020); potentially seasonal (Amani et al. 2020); believed to use a bat host (Hussain et al. 2020) and the relay host to humans could be mink (Faure and Sciama 2021), whose farms in China may exceed 100,000 per head – however the analysis of recombinations observed in SARS-CoV-2 does not yet provide any certainty about the interspecific links from which the virus originated (Liu et al. 2020). The symptoms of SARS-CoV-2 mainly affect the respiratory system and the elderly (in France, 75% of deaths involved people over 75 years of age), with a severity linked, in addition to the existence of comorbidities (present in 2 out of 3 victims), to a strong exacerbation of the inflammatory response (Émilie et al. 2020) and also to Kawasaki-like vascular damage in some children (Jones et al. 2020). Mortality associated with SARS-CoV-2, which mainly affects older people, is expected to result in only a moderate decline in average life expectancy, which in France is expected to be in the order of 0.2 to 0.6 years in 2020 (Guillot and Khiat 2020).

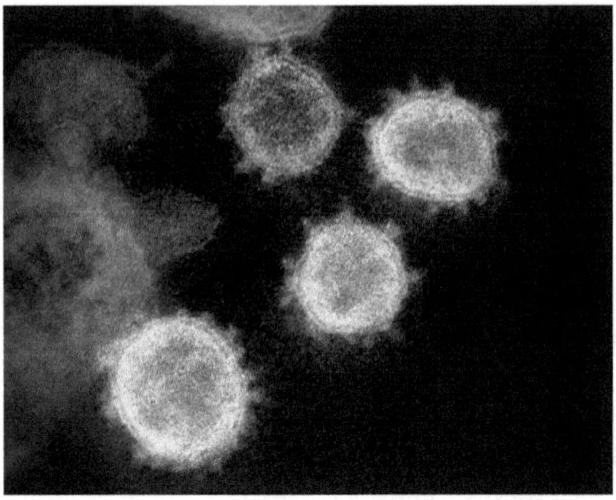

Figure 1.1. *SARS-CoV-2 viruses and their crown-shaped spicules, as seen by transmission electron microscopy (source: NIAID 2020)*

With regard to the prevention of epidemics and health crises – and based on France – the INRAE (*Institut national de recherche pour l'agriculture, l'alimentation et l'environnement*, National Research Institute for Agriculture, Food and the Environment) conducted a research program (EpiEmerge) in 2002–2004, within the framework of a conceptual reflection on epidemiological emergence, focusing on methods for studying emerging plant, animal and human diseases (Sache and Barnouin 2006); this was done using a conceptual approach that was at once biological, biomathematical, environmental, sociological and in terms of public management (Barnouin and Sache 2010). In addition, following the A/H1N1 influenza pandemic of 2009–2010, a national prevention and control plan, known as the *Pandémie grippale* (influenza pandemic), was established and subsequently revised in 2011 (SGD 2011); this plan constituted the reference for public authorities with regard to the Covid-19 crisis. In addition to the field of health and food safety, emerging technological risks are studied in France: at the École des Mines de Nantes by the chair "Emerging Risks and Technologies, from Technological Management to Social Regulation" (Guimard 2016), and in the nuclear safety and insurance sectors, via "risk barometers" (Chubb 2018). As for climate risks, they are monitored by the ONERC (*Observatoire national sur les effets du réchauffement climatique*, National Observatory on the Effects of Global Warming) (ONERC 2020). Despite these notable initiatives, significant progress seems to be required if we are to have, in France and elsewhere in the world, optimal operational capacities with regard to the harmful consequences of emerging risks on health.

The aim of this chapter is to draw lessons from the Covid-19 crisis, based on the history of the disease in France and its distribution throughout the world. Based on information disseminated by the authorities and the press, or from unpublished interviews with the actors of the epidemic, this work, which takes stock of the health crisis, is intended to be a combat tool for the fight against future emergencies.

1.1.2. *The emergence of the emergence*

1.1.2.1. *The facts*

The first three cases of Covid-19 were announced in France on January 24, 2020 by health authorities, while the first Chinese cases, reported in Wuhan (Hubei province), officially date from November 17, 2019, that is, 78 days before the first official French cases were announced.

The French cases concerned in particular a 48-year-old man from Bordeaux, of Chinese origin, who had traveled to Wuhan and Shanghai (China), returning to France on January 22 via the Bordeaux-Mérignac airfield (Gironde), and worked in the wine trade. The 40-year-old, who was treated at the Pellegrin hospital after consulting SOS Médecins, was released on February 13 after spending 22 days in quarantine. On leaving the Bordeaux University Hospital, the patient, a commercial intermediary between Bordeaux winegrowers and Chinese wishing to invest in wine estates, told a journalist:

> This forced isolation made me realize how precious daily life is. I was locked up. It was hard. That mundane, but fundamental freedom to be free to move, like going out on the street, going back and forth, is essential (Goinière 2020).

Previously, the salesman had stated, in reference to his hospitalization conditions at the Pellegrin University Hospital:

> Here, everyone who comes in is in a suit, with masks, gloves and glasses. We have no physical contact (Castera 2020).

The communicative inhabitant of Bordeaux, treated at the tropical and traveler diseases unit of the university hospital with the help of an antiviral, remdesivir (Cristiani 2020) – and who has since completely recovered from his infection – had moreover specified, speaking about China:

> At the beginning of last week, everyone knew that this virus existed, but people were not worried. In fact, very few people outside were wearing masks.

Believing that he was infected in the area of the Wuhan bus station, where the fish market is located and where the virus was reportedly detected – or even on the train – the patient stated: "I started coughing a few days later" (Castera 2020).

The other contaminations announced on January 24 concerned a Chinese couple, aged 30 and 31, from Wuhan, who arrived in Paris on January 18 and were treated at the Bichat hospital, from where they were discharged on February 12 (Mari 2020). In addition, an 81-year-old Chinese tourist from Hubei province, 400 km from Wuhan, who arrived in Paris on January 23 with his 50-year-old daughter, was diagnosed with the coronavirus on January 24 and hospitalized on January 25 at Bichat Hospital, where he died on January 28, becoming the first victim of Covid-19 in France and Europe. As for his daughter, she was cured after her stay at Bichat (France info

2020). One day after the Chinese tourist's death, Air France suspended its flights from Wuhan, with the destinations of Shanghai and Beijing being reduced in frequency from January 31 (Samama 2020).

In addition, a businessman from Servomex (a company specializing in gas analysis), who had just returned from Singapore where he had attended a conference at the Grand Hyatt hotel from January 21 to 23, went to the Contamines Montjoie ski resort in Haute-Savoie on January 24. He stayed there for four days, the time it took to infect five British people, including a child, who tested positive on February 8 and were hospitalized in Grenoble (Isère), Lyon (Rhône) and Saint-Étienne (Loire). The businessman then returned to England, where he was declared positive and was the source of at least five English cases, two of which were linked to doctors (Dugit 2020; Mc Lean and Feleke 2020), and of a cluster involving several municipalities in Haute-Savoie. During the conference organized by Servomex, a 27-year-old Singaporean contracted the virus via a conference employee living in Wuhan, and as a result, two South Koreans and a Malaysian tested positive on return to their countries (Mei and Taj 2020). In addition, the sequencing of SARS-CoV-2 by the Pasteur Institute was announced on January 29, and on January 30 the contamination of a Parisian doctor infected by Chinese patients who had left for Taiwan after having consulted him, a country in which one of them was declared infected (Mari 2020). January ended with the repatriation of Europeans living in Wuhan through the transport squadron 03.060 Estérel from Air Base 110 "Lieutenant-colonel Guy de La Horie" at Creil (Oise) (Ministère des Armées 2020b).

The history of initial cases of Covid-19 in France was called into question in May 2020 (Roy 2020). Indeed, a 42-year-old man living in Bondy (Seine-Saint-Denis), initially diagnosed with influenza on December 27, 2019, was recognized as suffering from Covid-19 on that date via analyses carried out a posteriori (the infected person's children also showed symptoms). The patient's wife, suspected asymptomatic, was declared to be in contact with Asian salesmen in her workplace. Other early cases were reported in Alsace via the hospital in Colmar (Haut-Rhin) on May 7: a 57-year-old man confirmed positive on December 2, 2019 and more than a dozen other cases – including two suspicions on November 16–17 and a suspect scan on November 1 (Haby 2020). As for a retrospective epidemiological study conducted on data from Haut-Rhin, it indicated that SARS-CoV-2 appeared to be circulating in this department as early as January (Gerbaud et al. 2020). In addition, French athletes who participated in the Military Games in Wuhan during the second half of October (the source of a Sino-American controversy on the possible epidemiological role of this event) (de Sèze 2020) believe that some of them were infected by Covid-19 following their stay in China, although their symptoms could not be validated as corresponding to this disease (Opoczinski 2020).

1.1.2.2. *Lessons learned*

The period from January 23 to February 1, 2020 corresponds to the epidemic peak of Covid-19 in China, essentially in Wuhan and Hubei, with an average of over 2,500 new cases per day (Wu and McGoogan 2020). There is then little doubt about the possible consequences of the viral emergence in France, which appears to be Wuhan-dependent, as confirmed by a sequencing study of SARS-CoV-2 conducted by the Pasteur Institute (Gámbaro 2020; Institut Pasteur 2020).

Furthermore, the first stage of the French emergence highlights, in addition to the risk of transmission via the Chinese epicenter of the epidemic, certain characteristics of the infection already observed in China: the significant contagiousness of the virus; a duration of a few days for incubation; greater involvement of men; severity in the elderly; the role of tourism and air transport; the risk for general practitioners; the effectiveness of strict isolation in preventing new contaminations; the tendency for initial underestimation of the danger of the epidemic and the acceleration of contagion by "congregated communities" comprising infected and non-sick – or unrecognized sick – individuals from various horizons who, on their return to their places of origin, could have been the agents of the outbreak or aggravation of a national epidemic – this being like the role played by the Metropole Hotel in Hong Kong (China) in the epidemic due to the SARS-CoV coronavirus (whose animal emergence chain may have involved the bat and the webbed civet), which caused nearly 900 deaths worldwide in 2002–2003 (Fraissard 2004). Thus, a probable health catastrophe was knocking on the door in France in the first phase of the epidemic.

In order to measure an emerging risk, it is necessary to have pre-positioned mobile teams capable of investigating, via legally enshrined intervention capacities, wherever the risk needs to be assessed. These teams must have investigative capabilities via dedicated logistics (servers, laboratory, means of transport) and varied skills. As we will see later, such an organization needs to be fully operational in order to control an emerging epidemic agent, in addition to the constitution of a multidisciplinary monitoring committee responsible for advising the State authorities. If such a committee appears to be indispensable, it seems nevertheless useful that it be composed of both confirmed experts and young innovative researchers, in order to be as informed and reactive as possible.

The type of organization mentioned above must allow for defensive measures to be taken that are as adapted as possible to an epidemic situation, following the infection as closely as possible, then overtaking it before "nipping it in the bud" by drying up its transmission. This type of organization requires that operational teams be linked to databases capable of self-modeling based on the current epidemic dynamics or even on those of previous epidemics. Since one of the conditions for successful infection control is the avoidance of contact and the protection of caregivers, the development of telemedicine and artificial intelligence, as well as the use of robots capable of performing certain medical procedures, should also be promoted in the initial epidemic phase (Saltmarsh 2020b). Nevertheless, the fact that the action of an emerging pathogen generally contains many gray areas may mean that the most appropriate decisions to counter its spread may not always be taken.

1.1.3. *Oise cluster*

1.1.3.1. *The facts*

On January 31, 193 Frenchmen were repatriated from Wuhan by the A340 of the Estérel squadron (Figure 1.2) from the Creil defence base (2,800 employees, including 800 civilians and 1,300 people assigned to military base 110). While Air Base 110 houses part of the military intelligence services – and should host the army's spy training center – its airstrip is hardly used anymore, which implies that the repatriation plane was stationed at the Roissy-Charles-de-Gaulle airport (Val-d'Oise), like the other planes of the squadron (assigned to military missions, transporting officials or repatriation) (Ministère des Armées 2018). The personnel of the Creil base, having taken charge of the flight to Wuhan, did not get off on arrival in China, the repatriated being, for their part, considered not sick, as they tested negative before boarding. Disembarking at Carry-le-Rouet (Bouches-du-Rhône) on their return to France, the repatriates remained in quarantine in closed buildings for 14 days and came out of the quarantine with no illness.

As for the about 15 colleagues from Air Base 110, they returned to their base after landing their aircraft at Roissy.

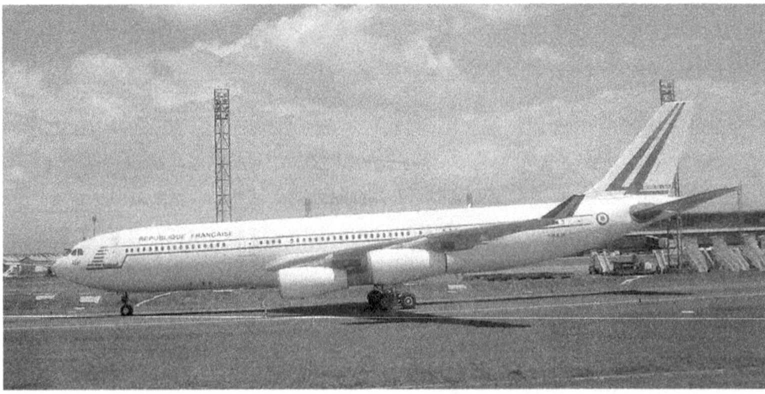

Figure 1.2. *Airbus A340 of the Estérel squadron (source: Mario Roberto Duran Ortiz Fabre, 2009)*

According to the Ministry of the Armed Forces, "upon return, the crew benefited from the surveillance protocol for 14 days spent at home, with temperature taken twice a day, and without having been tested by PCR (polymerase chain reaction) (Herrero 2020). After 14 days of monitoring, none showed any symptoms" (Ministère des Armées 2020a). A military source stated:

> None [of the officers who accompanied the returnees] was placed in quarantine, only on 14-day permission at their homes, but with no control over their whereabouts or those of their families (Gourru 2020a).

The base commander stated that the squadron members returning from China "did not have biological tests, but had regular check-ups during the incubation period and had not developed any symptoms since" (Gourru 2020b). It thus appears, unless we are mistaken, that the personnel of Air Base 110 were not subjected to a strict protocol of isolation in a closed environment and returned to live at home. As for the semi-quarantine applied to the Oise department, the first large-scale anti-Covid-19 measure adopted in France only began on March 1 (France info 2020b), that is, after the end of the period of supervised leave just mentioned and 105 days after the announcement of the first official Chinese cases.

A second plane, a chartered Airbus A380, repatriated 258 people on February 2 through the Estérel squadron, including 64 French people, 84 of whom were confined to Aix-en-Provence (Bouches-du-Rhône) after landing at the Istres base (France info 2020c). The strict quarantine – or lack thereof – of the personnel of the Creil base who ensured this flight was not identified, corresponding, as for the first repatriation, to a period in which no quarantine was carried out in the Oise. A dozen people – who were among those repatriated on February 2 – showed symptoms on arrival at Istres, which were not attributed to Covid-19, as these passengers tested negative. Some of the foreign nationals on board the A380 – 12 Belgians, 23 Dutch, 11 Danes, 5 Czechs and 2 Slovaks – then flew to Brussels. On arrival of the plane – on February 3 – at the Melsbroek military base, a Belgian passenger, following his admission to the Saint-Pierre hospital in Brussels, was recognized as suffering from Covid-19 (he was the first Belgian to be recognized as infected). This passenger was kept in isolation in hospital until February 15, like the 11 other asymptomatic passengers (France info 2020d; RTBF Info 2020).

According to the Ministry of the Armed Forces,

> A third rotation via the military base of Istres (Bouches-du-Rhône) was carried out on February 9. CBRN (chemical, biological, radiological and nuclear defense) experts from the military air expertise center, as well as CBRN-E teams from BA 120 in Cazaux (Gironde), were then mobilized to ensure the disinfection of the plane (a Boeing 747-400 chartered by the British authorities) and of the means of transporting the passengers, with the support of the air force firefighters from Air Base 115 in Orange (Vaucluse) and 125 in Istres (Ministère des Armées 2020b).

The 35 French passengers of the Boeing, which had carried a total of 200 people, most of them British citizens, had transited through Brize Norton airfield (Oxfordshire), before reaching the Istres base and being placed in quarantine in Aix-en-Provence. One of these passengers, who was suffering, was temporarily transferred to the Méditerranée Infection University Hospital Institute in Marseille (Bouches-du-Rhône) to undergo tests for SARS-CoV-2, which proved to be negative (Vergnenère 2020). In addition, 64 repatriates living in Wuhan landed at Roissy-Charles-de-Gaulle on February 21 in a chartered A380, including 28 French nationals who were directed to Branville (Calvados) to be quarantined there for 14 days (France info 2020e).

Following these risky repatriations, two cases of Covid-19 appeared in the Oise region: a 55-year-old man, a bus driver at Air Base 110 in Creil (35,000 inhabitants) and residing in La Croix-Saint-Ouen (4,300 inhabitants); and a 60-year-old man, a technology teacher at the Jean de la Fontaine high school in Crépy-en-Valois (15,000 inhabitants) and residing in Vaumoise (1,000 inhabitants) (La Croix 2020a). The living environments of these two contaminants were very close, with 31 km and 26 km separating their workplaces, on the one hand, and their homes, on the other hand (Figure 1.3). The driver, following the appearance of symptoms on February 12–13, was hospitalized (on the 16th?) in Compiègne and admitted to the intensive care unit on February 18 (a unit that was then temporarily closed), before being transferred on February 22 to the university hospital in Amiens ("where other patients suspected of being affected had been admitted") following the worsening of his condition (Coq-Chodorge 2020).

At Compiègne hospital, the driver's illness was not immediately identified, and the patient had time to come into contact with 117 people before being recognized as Covid-positive, with 20 suspected carers being sent home as a result (Julien 2020a). The teacher, on sick leave from February 12, was sent to Creil hospital (whose intensive care unit was closed after his visit and where agents were quarantined). He stayed there from February 19 to 25, before being transferred to the Pitié-Salpêtrière Hospital and dying there on the night of February 25 (La Croix 2020a).

If the information we have been able to access is accurate, we can see that the driver's and the teacher's symptoms started at the same period (within two to three days), with contaminations having to occur between February 4 and 8. At these dates, the Chinese outbreak was by far the most active, even though two Chinese tourists had been diagnosed with Covid-19 as early as January 30 in Milan (Le Parisien 2020a). Moreover, while the teacher had no history of contact with China or Italy, the driver was part of the professional community (Air Base 110) whose teams repatriated a large number of people living in Wuhan, the heart of the Chinese epidemic; teams that stayed on February 2 (and before February 2, on January 31) for nearly 11 hours in a plane with repatriated Europeans, at least one of whom was found to be infected with SARS-CoV-2 upon arrival in Brussels.

Thus, assuming that a crew member at Air Base 110 was infected on January 31 or February 2, he could have infected the driver (and others on the base) around February 6–8. In this regard, the driver's wife stated that her husband had been in contact with, among others, the husband of a (possibly asymptomatically infected) flight attendant on the January 31 repatriation plane (Julien 2020b). It is important at this point to note that 20–50% of SARS-CoV-2 transmissions are linked to asymptomatic carriers (a study conducted in the educational community of the Crépy-en-Valois high school put the proportion at 17%) (Fontanet et al. 2020).

It is to be noted that the epidemiological significance of asymptomatic infected people implies that the absence of clinical cases, as was the case for personnel on repatriation flights, is not synonymous with the certainty of non-infection, as a proportion of these officials, although not recognized as infected, may have in fact been infected (testing for the presence of SARS-CoV-2 is not sensitive if the patient is not in the acute sympathetic phase or if the viral load is low, and serological tests are not recommended during the first week of the onset of symptoms) (Haute autorité de santé 2020).

Although an epidemiological investigation refuted it (Ministère des Armées 2020a), a rather probable hypothesis, with regard to the formation of the Oise cluster, concerns transmission of SARS-CoV-2 by asymptomatic (or very weakly symptomatic) contaminated personnel of Air Base 110. These personnel were not strictly quarantined and not tested (Herrero 2020) following their missions in China, and could have been the source of transmissions directly to colleagues at the air base, such as the driver, and indirectly, to people outside the base through "their life after the repatriation flights" in Crépy-en-Valois, Creil, Compiègne or elsewhere, despite certain precautions taken within Air Base 110 (Courrier picard 2020a). In any case, the personnel of the base were significantly affected by Covid-19, following the infection of the driver. Thus, the *Courrier picard* of March 16, representing *Agence France-Presse*, indicated that 16 people working at base 110 had tested positive for SARS-CoV-2 and that two had been hospitalized (Courrier picard 2020a). As for the epidemiological link between "Air Base 110" and "the teacher", it probably originated from contact, in the days following the repatriations, between the teacher – through a member of his very close entourage – and one or more members of the personnel of Air Base 110.

The Oise cluster, in addition to having generated victims, was at the origin of secondary outbreaks in their places of residence (thus, on March 1, a 39-year-old employee of the Creil base living in Pas-de-Calais was recognized as infected and inaugurated the contamination of this department), including overseas (a couple living on the Caribbean island of Saint-Martin, following a stay in Oise, was declared positive on February 29) (BFM TV 2020). The Oise cluster involved communal groupings, notably in Crépy-en-Valois, with seven people dead as of March 7, including four in the EHPAD (*Établissement d'hébergement pour personnes âgées dépendantes*, Establishment for the Accommodation of Dependent Elderly Citizens) (Courrier picard 2020b). Crépy-en-Valois was also the place of residence of the third French death linked to Covid-19, in this case an 89-year-old woman who died in the hospital in Compiègne during the night of February 29 (France info 2020f).

A gateway for the virus to enter Oise, apart from repatriations, could have been linked to staff at Roissy-Charles-de-Gaulle airport, via flights from China or even Italy. Indeed, 18% of the 90,000 people working in connection with Roissy live in the Oise, according to a study by R'Pro'Mobilité (2016). Thus, nearly 250 employees linked to Roissy-Charles-de-Gaulle live in Crépy-en-Valois, and nearly 150 in Chantilly and Compiègne. Nevertheless, 21% of these employees live in Seine-et-Marne, which is the Île-de-France department most spared from Covid-19 (mortality is 14 times lower there than in Oise).

As for the airport staff, including those of Air France, they were seemingly spared by the virus, even though on February 27, a temporary worker who had worked at Roissy "a few weeks" before being recognized as infected was announced to have been infected by the coronavirus: "There could not therefore have been any transmission in this context", indicated the prefecture of Val-d'Oise on February 28 (Dutheil 2020). Nevertheless, airport staff or asymptomatic travelers returning from China or Italy – and having stayed in the "epidemic triangle" (Figure 1.3) – may have contributed to the initiation of viral circulation in the Oise region, although there is no evidence to support this hypothesis. Note that, at the beginning of March, the French General Directorate of Health estimated that 76% of Covid-19 cases whose origin of transmission had been elucidated were most likely linked to chain transmissions within the national territory, probably mainly in the Oise region; and that 26% were linked to transmissions originating from tourists or professionals who had arrived from countries affected by the pandemic, such as China or Italy.

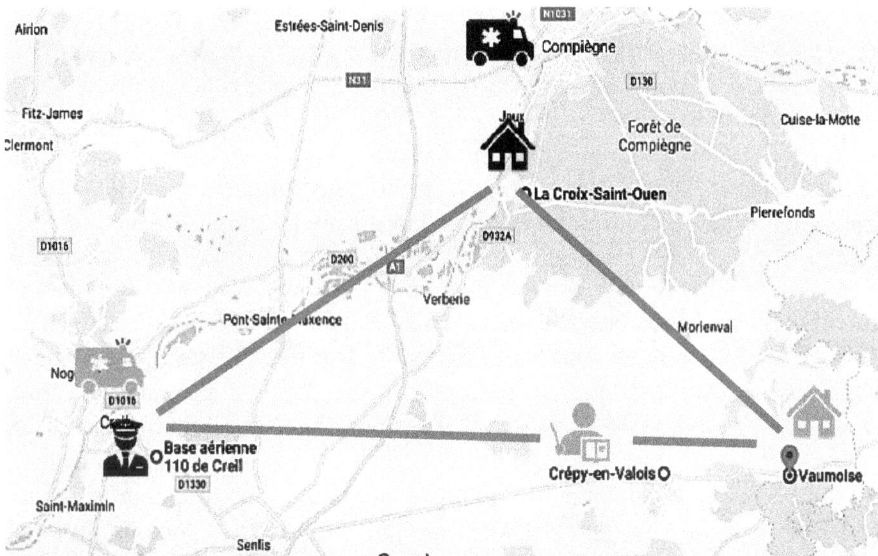

Figure 1.3. *"Epidemic triangle" in the Oise region (places of work, residence and hospitalization: Creil air base driver, in green; Crépy-en-Valois high school teacher, in black) (source: J. Barnouin, based on Google Maps, cartographic data ©2020 Google)*

1.1.3.2. *Lessons learned*

The constitution of the Oise cluster points to the role of epidemic exacerbation of groups (professional, social, etc.), through the 110 military base and the EHPAD. The non-existence of a global analysis methodology of the epidemic (from field investigation to modeling, including screening) based on the early dynamics of the French cases, with reference to documented epidemics and to the cases observed in Hubei (if, at least, the distribution of the cases disclosed by the Chinese authorities corresponds to the reality of the epidemic), probably did not help in measuring the danger and establishing in the best possible way the quarantining of the population and the ban on gatherings.

Moreover, French society as a whole was not sufficiently aware, in the early days of the epidemic, of the barrier measures that could counter a virus and of the rigor with which it was necessary to apply infection control measures. However, the French population – and the citizens of many nations – were faced with a poorly known threat, which their collective unconscious did not believe would happen other than in a disaster movie, and which did not seem to concern them, but only distant countries more or less suspected of non-transparency or laxity. Also, a certain optimism and a certain excessive belief in the strength of democratic motivations and a libertarian art of living reigned in French society and other equivalent societies, as if such societal traits could constitute an antidote to the contamination by a very contagious virus and its deleterious effects.

Although France did not have a pre-positioned system dedicated to emerging diseases before the crisis, INRAE had nevertheless designed in 2008, in collaboration with the Sciensano Institute (Brussels) and as a follow-up to the EpiEmerge program mentioned above, a real-time detection system for atypical syndromes applicable to animals and humans (Barnouin 2009a). However, this system, whose characteristics will be specified later, had not been implemented at all in France and had not obtained, in Belgium, the funds necessary for its permanent implementation (this was the problem encountered in France with surgical masks, whose stocks, expensive to maintain in "normal times", were not sufficiently abundant when the Covid-19 epidemic broke out).

The emergence of Covid-19 shows how interesting it would be to have maps of risk areas adapted to the various types of emergence. In this respect, the Val-d'Oise and Oise should be considered first and foremost and should probably be developed specifically. The elements to be considered in this area concern first of all the presence of a major international airport, Roissy-Charles-de-Gaulle, notably its links with China. Roissy is said to be the most exposed airport in the Western world to Covid-19, ahead of San Francisco, Los Angeles and Melbourne (Gardner et al. 2020). Another airport, Beauvais (Oise), is very active towards the Italian risk zone, with routes (suspended on March 8) to Bologna, Milan and Venice; and Paris-Le Bourget airport (Seine-Saint-Denis) is the leading *business* airport in Europe, with the Creil base being, as we have seen, in the front line for emergency air missions. The proximity of Paris and the fact that its region has 12.2 million inhabitants (1,000 inhabitants/km^2) are also characteristics to be considered in a global anti-epidemic prevention. In this context, the professional and personal relationships between places, companies and personnel working in air transport should also be taken into account in order to establish general preventive measures or measures applicable in times of crisis.

1.1.4. *The Haut-Rhin and the Grand Est mega-cluster*

1.1.4.1. *The facts*

On February 27, new cases of Covid-19 were reported concerning, in addition to a 33-year-old French–Chinese woman who had returned to Paris from China on February 7: a 64-year-old French man who had enjoyed repeated stays in Lombardy, hospitalized in Annecy (Haute-Savoie), and whose wife also tested positive, as did his daughter and a friend; a 50-year-old man hospitalized in Lyon (Rhône) who had not been to China or Italy (Bouhaut and Rosique 2020); and a 36-year-old French man back from Milan and identified in Strasbourg (Bas-Rhin) on February 25, who then became the "first" Covid-positive person in the Alsace region (Sud-Ouest 2020). On March 1, this man's partner, aged 32, was identified as being infected, as well as a 27-year-old woman and her children (1 and 5 years old), hospitalized in Strasbourg and living in the Haut-Rhin region (Préfecture du Haut-Rhin 2020); and on March 6, it was learned that, out of the 16 cases now confirmed in Alsace, 7 were linked to a religious gathering. Then, this number gradually increased, 18 of the relatives of the organizer of the gathering being contaminated, before accelerating again.

Thus, on March 23, 693 people affected by Covid-19 were hospitalized in the Haut-Rhin, including 162 hospital deaths (Préfecture du Haut-Rhin 2020), and the department became the main French epidemic focus. The outbreak quickly spread to the Grand Est region, the Lyon region and everywhere else, including Guyana (five cases) and Lot-et-Garonne (two cases). On her own, a nurse at the Strasbourg University Hospital – having attended the religious gathering in Mulhouse – could have contaminated 250 caregivers (Yahoo! Actualités 2020). As the situation worsened in the Haut-Rhin cluster, with hospitals on the verge of collapse and exhausted caregivers, serious cases were being moved by *TGV sanitaires* (high-speed train) or by air, towards areas little affected by the epidemic process.

Before the epidemic situation in the Haut-Rhin and the Grand Est region took off, a religious gathering (Figure 1.4) was held from February 17 to 21 (some people stayed until the 23rd) in Mulhouse (Haut-Rhin), an urban area of 290,000 inhabitants. This gathering was organized by the *Porte ouverte chrétienne* (the PO), an evangelical charismatic church preaching healing, salvation of souls and evangelization, and attracting evangelical Protestants and former Catholics, mainly from working-class backgrounds in the eastern departments (Jova 2020).

The Mulhouse gathering was a week of fasting and prayer shared by perhaps 2,500 people in a confined area (gatherings of more than 1,000 people were only banned in France from March 8). The week of spiritual exchange was free to attend and scheduled each day from 9:30 a.m. to 1:30 p.m. and from 5:00 p.m. to 9:30 p.m. (that is more than 40 hours of living together). "We spent a week praying together", said a PO pastor, "holding hands, kissing. We were not aware of what was going on" (Jova 2020). In short, as France Bleu radio put it:

> Close and repeated contact between people from all over France and the French overseas territories creates an ideal situation for spreading a virus…

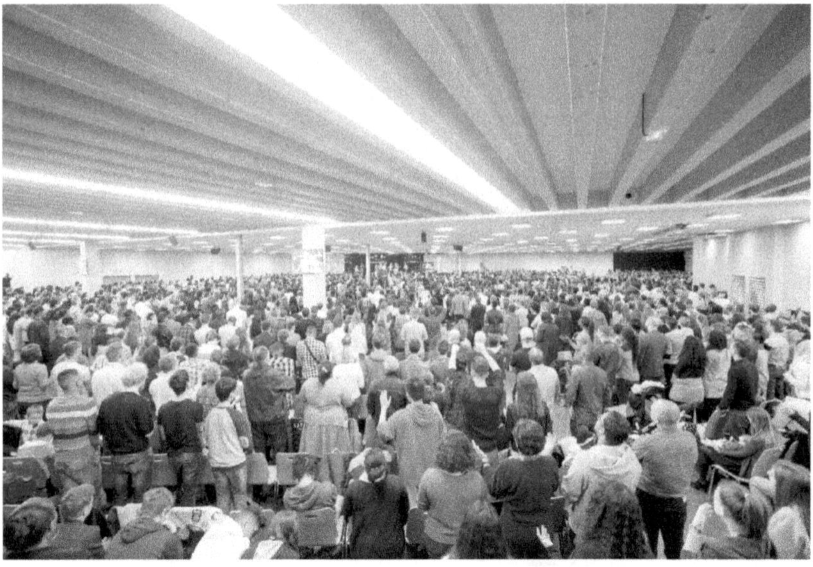

Figure 1.4. *Worship at the* Porte ouverte chrétienne *(Mulhouse, Haut-Rhin) (source: Porte ouverte chrétienne and Nathalieschnoebelen 2017)*

The high point of the gathering was the mass on Sunday February 23, which was held, like the rest of the week, in a former supermarket in the working-class district of Bourtzwiller, transformed into a place of worship. "We are unable to say exactly how many people are affected. Dozens and dozens…", confessed the pastor of the *Porte ouverte chrétienne*. As he explained, there were no lists of participants and no registrations. The faithful came for one or two days, or for an evening, before returning to their homes in France and neighboring countries, such as Switzerland. "It's very, very variable", he added. One participant believed that the number of 2,200 participants (including 300 children) could be underestimated, as some of the faithful came and went throughout the week. One thing was certain, however: everyone came by individual means and there was no chartered bus (Costentin and Genton 2020).

A large gathering, many contacts over a long period of time in a confined atmosphere, groups coming from many directions and returning, all the elements were present for this gathering to be synonymous, from the virus' point of view, with beneficial dissemination. An assessment made through the contacts of a participant at the meeting indicated that at least 75% of the participants at the meeting could have been clinically infected. As for the organizer of this meeting, to explain his low awareness of the epidemic risk, he stated:

> On Tuesday, February 18, the President of the Republic was there, 300 meters from the church, shaking hands with people, recalls the pastor. There was no barrier, no precautionary measures. We cannot be blamed for not having taken measures, for the simple reason that they did not exist.

Then the pastor reminded us:

> At the end of our gathering, there was still no chain of contamination in France, according to the *Agence nationale de la santé* [French National Health Agency]. The agency called us on March 1, because a mother whose children had come to our gathering had tested positive for coronavirus. We gave them all the addresses and contacts, put her calls on our website and immediately suspended our services. We did not hide anything (Le Parisien 2020b).

Moreover, according to the organizers of the evangelical week, none of the participants in the gathering had shown "signs of influenza" (Le Parisien 2020c), a statement that may be linked to the activity report, which was probably silent on this point, of the meeting's first aid service.

Where did the *Porte ouverte* contamination come from? It should have been due either to participants coming or returning from Italy or the Oise region (the main French epidemic cluster in mid-February), or to a local circulation through people coming from the Chinese epidemic focus. First element of reflection: the first Alsatian case of infection "outside the *Porte ouverte* gathering" was for a long time considered to be due to a man who returned from Milan on February 25, that is, 8 days after the beginning of the Mulhouse gathering (Sud-Ouest 2020)[1]. Namely, the first death attributed to date to Covid-19 in Northern Italy, which concerned – on February 21 – a 78-year-old man living in Veneto (de Filippis 2020).

In addition, researchers at the Sacco Hospital (Milan) isolated around February 15 the "Italian version" of the coronavirus, which "had been circulating unnoticed for weeks in the peninsula. The virus had been present for a long time, perhaps even before mid-January", as the hospital director said. According to this professional, the version of SARS-CoV-2 most present in Italy "was the result of a mutation, especially since this virus can change from person to person" (Le Parisien 2020d). While this statement does not seem to have been confirmed since, the high mortality rate due to Covid-19 in Italy is a cause for concern. The fact that the Italian population is the oldest in the world – after that of Japan – could be a factor explaining the severity of the epidemic in Italy. Nevertheless, Japan is one of the countries that has been little affected by the pandemic. However, the stereotypical characteristics of the Japanese, the second earliest non-Chinese population infected with SARS-CoV-2 after that of Thailand, are that they "don't touch", keep their distance and are disciplined (characteristics that are not shared by the Italians or French). Thus, distancing could be, in the first analysis, one of the predominant factors of the risk of contamination by SARS-CoV-2 (as of April 23, 2020, there were 299 deaths attributed in Japan to the pandemic coronavirus, against 21,340 in France and 25,085 in Italy; as well as 4,632 in China and 43 in Cameroon). Of course, these figures have changed significantly since then, with about 19,000 deaths in Japan, 4,700 in China and 1,600 in Cameroon as of October 2021, compared to more than 131,000 in Italy and 117,000 in France. Nevertheless, these developments do not call into question the major differences mentioned above. As for the care of the elderly in Asian countries, and in particular in Japan, they are almost entirely the responsibility of families, unlike in certain European countries, where many elderly people (750,000 in France, average

1 This case is no longer the original Alsatian case at all.

age 85) attend or live in retirement homes, which are riskier places than the family home in terms of contamination (accumulation of people at risk and large number of visitors).

Let us return to Mulhouse. Another element concerning the possible Italy–Mulhouse link, with regard to the SARS-CoV-2 contamination of the participants in the *Porte ouverte* gathering, was confirmed by an interview with the president of SOS Médecins 68. This general practitioner, contacted for the purposes of this study, indicated that he had witnessed the first suspected cases in connection with the evangelical gathering on February 24 and 25, 2020, through the members of two families who had been in contact with Italians "who were coughing and had a fever" during the gathering (Pietri 2020).

The investigation we carried out among the participants in the gathering confirmed the presence at the ceremony of an Italian family, which had moreover specified its nationality when the pastor questioned the faithful about their origin. It is therefore likely that a major source of contamination of the evangelicals gathered in Mulhouse, only 375 km from Milan, could have been of Italian origin. It could have been either direct or indirect (both modalities could have come into play), through the circulation of SARS-CoV-2 which seems to have affected Alsace since November 2019 (Haby 2020), a circulation possibly linked, hypothesis to be confirmed, to Chinese tourism. Colmar, a city of 70,000 inhabitants in the Haut-Rhin, is indeed very well known in China following the production in the Alsatian city of a season of the famous Chinese reality show *Chinese Restaurant*, broadcast from July 20, 2018.

In addition to Italy, Oise could have been involved in the transmission of the virus in Mulhouse. Indeed, the driver of the Creil base mentioned above was hospitalized in Compiègne on February 12, while the departure of the three (only) inhabitants of Oise (two from Compiègne and one from Senlis), aged about 60, who went to the Mulhouse gathering according to our investigation, dates from February 16, a period when the transmission chain was already active in Oise. One of these people, who tested positive for SARS-CoV-2 after returning from Mulhouse (as did the other two people from Isère), said:

> I went home on Friday night [21]. On Sunday [23], I was not very well. And then on Monday [24], I started to have a fever. I

> thought I had the flu. I was in bed for 11 days. A doctor friend of mine said: no, but that's too long. It can't be the flu. I was really weak. I couldn't even walk up three flights of stairs. Paramedics came to get me at my home and I was hospitalized for four days in Compiègne (Dargnies 2020).

Insofar as none of the three people from Isère who came to the Mulhouse gathering were ill or suspected of having Covid-19 before their departure, that none of them knew anyone infected in the Oise region and that all of them came back infected after the gathering (with symptoms appearing seven to nine days after the beginning of the event, and therefore compatible with an infection that took place at the beginning of the evangelical week), infection of the *Porte ouverte* gathering – via the circulation of the virus in the Oise cluster – thus appears unlikely; thus, the Isariens (the inhabitants of Oise) were probably infected in Mulhouse.

This raises the question of viral strains (Tan et al. 2020a), discussed in relation to Italy, or rather that of viral isolates linked to mutations or RNA copy errors. These are extremely frequent in coronavirus (of the order of 10^5 to 10^6 times every 6 hours) (Martin 2020b), while corresponding to mutations that do not usually lead to a change in virulence. However, if SARS-CoV-2 mutations are not silent, they can lead to an increase in the contagiousness of the virus and a reduction in its virulence (Korber et al. 2020). Could Mulhouse have been an evolutionary laboratory for the virus, as well as an epidemiological kettle? A study of the viral variants (one variant differs from another by very slight genetic differences, whereas the strains have much more significant differences between them) that have circulated in Alsace will perhaps be produced one day, which could explain more precisely the formation of the Grand Est mega-cluster from contamination by the variants that caused the very high incidence and mortality observed around Bergamo and Milan.

1.1.4.2. *Lessons learned*

The formation of the Haut-Rhin cluster indicates that in the preventive control of an epidemic threat, the management of groups and gatherings is fundamental, as is social distancing. The Mulhouse gathering, with its hugs, embraces and hand holdings, was thus a kind of model in terms of risk, as has been argued above, in contrast to the cultural practices of distancing of the Japanese. In Japan, the bow, which is known to Europeans through judo, is governed by codes inculcated from an early age. The bow is a sign of consideration for the person with whom they are dealing and has several meanings, depending on the context and the degree of bowing: a simple, quick nod, an expression of thanks or apology, as well as a way of asserting social position.

A few uncontrolled gatherings – occurring during the diffusion phase of a highly contagious pathogen – can have a considerable impact on the severity of an epidemic. This issue has been raised in particular in Italy in relation to coronavirus, with reference to a Champions League football match held on February 19, 2020, in Milan between the teams Atalanta Bergamo and Valencia (Tanguy 2020b) (Figure 1.5). This match gathered 45,000 spectators, several thousands of whom were from Spain, with thousands of tifosi also gathered in bars and restaurants in Bergamo to enjoy the event. Thus, the match may have been a significant factor in the spread of the coronavirus in northern Italy – and particularly in Bergamo, a city of 120,000 inhabitants located 60 km from Milan (1.4 million inhabitants). In this city, considered as "the Italian Wuhan", we do not understand why such a high mortality rate, which at one point concerned more than 9% of the patients, was observed, while the area is renowned for the quality of its health system (Dupont 2020). It is therefore difficult not to wonder whether viral isolates with high pathogenicity impacted this region. Following the Bergamo–Valencia match on February 19, it should be noted that 35% of the Valencia team's players and coaches were found to be Covid-positive, although no serious cases were reported among these athletes, the vast majority of whom were young (L'Équipe 2020).

The same questioning that has shaken Italy has arisen in France concerning a Lyon–Juventus match that brought together 40,000 French and Italian fans 15 km from Lyon on February 26, 2020, a match in which thousands of fans spread out in the streets of "the capital of Gauls" and on the stadium grounds (Faure 2020).

On the other hand, in Spain, the role of demonstrations, such as the one that brought together 120,000 people in Madrid on March 8 – on the occasion of International Women's Day – was questioned in relation to the spread of the Covid-19 epidemic (due to the number of people, the low level of distancing, the direct contacts and the chanting of slogans). The seriousness of the epidemic was not necessarily recognized at the time in the Iberian peninsula, if we refer to the slogans of the rally, one of which stated:

"machismo kills more than the coronavirus" (La Croix 2020b). As mentioned above, we are touching here on a certain unconsciousness of prosperous Western societies, proud of their freedom of opinion and morals, with regard to a threat that does not seem to concern them, as if democracy and unhindered expression protected them from emerging viral threats.

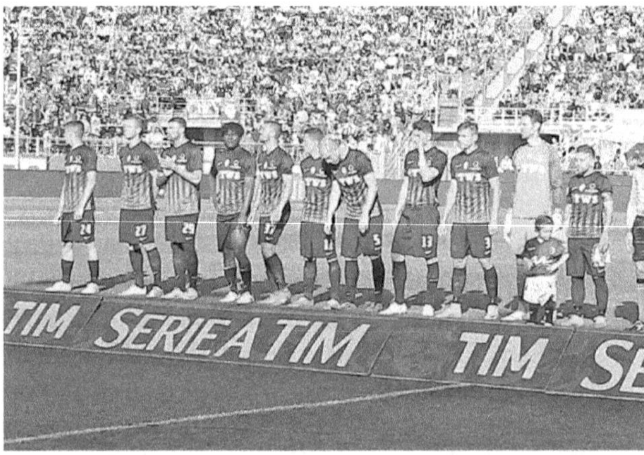

Figure 1.5. *View of the Bergamo stadium where the Atalanta Bergamo–Valencia match took place on February 19, 2020 (source: Save the Dream 2017)*

The question of the epidemiological role of gatherings and their prohibition, as measures to limit the epidemic risk, could only benefit from modeling. Indeed, modeling would help to make decision-making more reliable by considering, in the Covid-19 risk associated with gatherings, the weight of all the risk factors, that is, the number and dynamics of participants; the contagiousness parameters of the virus; the duration of contact and the contact conditions associated with the gathering; the participants' return journeys; the estimated rate of infection at the beginning of the gathering; and the level of infection in the general population and/or the region concerned by the gathering. All of this implies that in "alert periods", gathering organizers should be required to declare their gatherings, request permission to hold them, transmit lists of registrants and their addresses and discourage the attendance of tired or ill people.

Generally speaking, when it comes to deciding on the application of barrier measures in relation to a risk of contamination by an emerging virus in a naive population, the two decision-making paths are: a statistical path, based on probabilities, in particular through methods adapted to rare events and spatio-temporal variables (Barnouin and Sache 2010); and an observational path, based on the observation of specific facts, the occurrence of which almost automatically triggers population protection measures. In the case of the Covid-19 epidemic that affected France, a certain number of observations and facts could have led to a strict lockdown of the population, with however a delay of one week between the announcement of the lockdown decision and the lockdown itself, with the aim of preparing people's minds and the management system.

These observations and facts are:

1) the announcement of the first three cases diagnosed on the national territory, which could have led to a lockdown on January 31;

2) the contamination of an employee of a sensitive work community (Air Base 110), which could have led to a lockdown on February 19;

3) the observation that a chain of contamination was likely to have been established in a high-risk region, which could have been the basis for a lockdown from February 26 onwards;

4) the death of a French man in France who was contaminated, which could have resulted in a lockdown on March 3;

5) the observation of the 30th death on the national territory, which could have led to the lockdown of the French population on March 13.

In practice, lockdown, which the Pasteur Institute confirms was effective against Covid-19 (Salje et al. 2020a), was implemented in France from March 17, which appears to have been far too late, even though quarantine had prevented between 1,000 and 4,800 deaths by March 31, according to modeling conducted at Imperial College (Flaxman et al. 2020). Nevertheless, the French authorities were faced with an unprecedented health crisis that they managed "as best they could" in a nation divided and suspicious of its elites, which might have entered into acute agitation had early, yet beneficial, containment been instituted. The crisis was also unprecedented, as it was caused by an infectious agent that was poorly known, more contagious than expected and difficult to treat, and it had uncertain consequences at the national and international levels. It was also not possible to resolve it early with the help of a real-time monitoring system for epidemiological emergencies, as this did not exist (and still does not exist) in France and elsewhere, as will be presented in the following section.

In analyzing the potential consequences of the five key dates proposed above, we find that:

– the date of lockdown number 1, January 31, would have offerred partial protection from the consequences of the large clusters of infection in Oise and complete protection from the "mega-cluster" of the Haut-Rhin (hence a modest epidemic);

– date number 2, that is, February 19 (which would have been announced on the 12th), would not have protected against the Oise clusters, but would against that of the Haut-Rhin (hence a moderate epidemic);

– date number 3, February 26, would not have protected against the start-up of these two clusters but would probably have significantly limited the consequences of the Haut-Rhin cluster and therefore the mortality;

– date number 4, March 3, would have limited in part the consequences of the Haut-Rhin cluster;

– date number 5, March 13, would have decreased the overall impact of the epidemic compared to what was experienced, but not by much.

We conclude from this first analysis that a general lockdown of France (without applying it to vital or strategic activities) should have been announced on February 12 at the latest, with an effective start on February 19 (as a consequence of the damage to a sensitive work community), that is, 29 days before the lockdown as it was actually implemented. It should be noted that the choice of this date would have led, inter alia, to the postponement of the municipal elections (against which the French political parties were vehemently opposed) and the cancellation of the Lyon–Juventus match (which would also have led to very negative reactions). Nevertheless, it should be specified that the present reflection, carried out in the midst of the epidemic's development, if it can indicate the general ways of anti-epidemic's protection which would have to be followed, is not able to establish precise observations on the health and economic consequences of a decision of early lockdown, consequences whose evaluation can only result from modeling which must have, to be relevant, all the data and information available, once the crisis has come to an end.

Another point of criticism in the management of the beginning of the crisis in France, a delicate moment when the risk was still not fully appreciated, was the fact that the transport of the returnees from the Chinese epidemic was supervised by personnel from a professional community of 1,300 people (or even 2,500, if we refer to the whole of the defense base), a large community in which these personnel returned from China without having been, it seems, strictly isolated. This was an imprudent way of acting, and perhaps the door through which, at least according to one hypothesis, "the wolf of Wuhan entered the Isarian sheepfold".

1.2. Characteristics of an outbreak control system that could potentially control Covid-19

1.2.1. *Detection of the atypical and the bizarre*

The Covid-19 crisis raises many questions, in addition to those addressed in the deciphering of the epidemic, including in particular the issue of controlling wildlife and pathogens common to both animals and humans (Barnouin 2004) (Figure 1.6). The ceasing of any practice leading, by will of profit, ignorance or tradition, to the bringing together of human populations and wild animals – via contact, consumption or fetishism – thus appears to be an absolute necessity, considering in particular the conditions of emergence that seem to have presided, according to the current hypotheses, over the diffusion of the coronavirus pandemic towards humans (Liu et al. 2020).

Thus, the study of wild hosts (Mandl et al. 2020) of bacteria, viruses and other parasites, and the question of the conditions for crossing the species barrier (Barnouin and Sache 2010; Barnouin 2012), should have a bright future in terms of research and health management (see the ZooCov project developed at the *Centre de coopération internationale en recherche agronomique pour le développement* (CIRAD, French Agricultural Research Centre for International Development)). This question implies the need for humanity to organize, in a generic manner, a questioning of the place of wild animals, and in particular of wild species raised (Faure and Sciama 2021) for food, fur or magical beliefs. The question of epidemics should not be considered strictly from the point of view of the pathogenicity of infectious agents, but also from the point of view of the "environmental aggressiveness" that humans deploy as the dominant species. We can therefore see that the question of the emergence of a human disease cannot be detached from the general ecology of infectious agents, particularly through the relations between animal diseases and human diseases, which appear to be involved in the main recent health crises (acquired immunodeficiency syndrome (AIDS), bovine spongiform encephalopathy (BSE), influenza A/H1N1, coronavirus infections) (Faure and Sciama 2021).

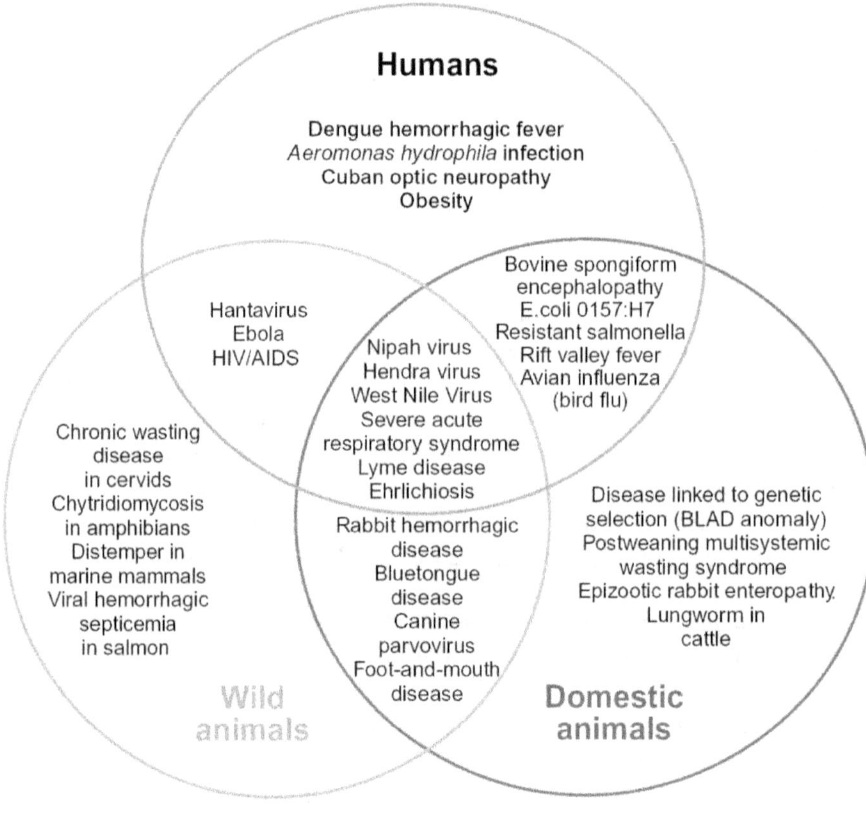

Figure 1.6. *Diseases located at the crossroads of wild animals, domestic animals and humans (Barnouin and Vourc'h 2004)*

Emerging diseases are disease processes that include clinical and/or epidemiological patterns that do not correspond to a known disease, or appear to correspond to a known disease in an unusual or unexpected form, in terms of the species or type of affected individual, severity, area of occurrence or non-response to usually effective treatment (Barnouin and Sache 2010). Emergence also corresponds to a significant increase in the number of cases of a known disease in an area where it was expected, a problem corresponding to that of the existence of localized emergences within an endemic disease (Barnouin and Sache 2010), such as seasonal influenza.

Detecting the unexpected, the bizarre, the unusual, the unknown and the worrisome requires the development of analysis systems different from those used to monitor listed diseases (Abat et al. 2016). Detecting the unknown and the potentially dangerous implies early analysis and rapid decision-making, in order to stop an emergence with epidemic or even pandemic potential. To do this, an anti-epidemic system is needed: pre-positioned, permanent, agile, rapid, open, with decision rules adapted to the main epidemic scenarios and linked to the decision-making authority, that is, if we act at the national level (the simplest and most operational to achieve), at the highest governmental level. The national level must be coupled with an international cooperation with the ambition of setting up, if possible, a universal network for the detection of emerging syndromes. Finally, an epidemic prevention system is closer to the mindset of a terrorist threat detection unit than to that of a traditional disease surveillance structure.

The major factors of epidemiological emergence concern humans, animals and plants:

a) the ecology of infectious agents, via untimely comparisons between species (e.g. a chimpanzee infected with a virus and a human being to whom this virus is transmitted during a hunt, following a bite, a graze or the consumption of the monkey's meat: case of AIDS);

b) carelessness relating to industrial food (case of BSE and animal meal), trade (import–export of contaminated plants) and the escape of pathogenic strains from a biology laboratory (see the hypotheses put forward and rejected concerning the involvement of the P4 laboratory ("class 4 pathogen") of the Wuhan Institute of Virology in the initiation of Covid-19, via the escape of a SARS-CoV-2 strain from this laboratory) (Bacqué and Pedroletti 2020);

c) agro-bio-terrorist activities that could be conducted for economic warfare purposes, through a major food source, such as wheat (Barnouin and Sache 2010);

d) economic crises disrupting the nutritional balance of populations and inducing pathologies – with an epidemic appearance – with a nutritional component, such as the epidemic neuropathy that occurred in Cuba in the 1990s (Barnouin 2001; de Sèze 2020).

Hence the need to set up specific prepositioned organizations aimed at early containment of epidemiological outbreaks or even preventing them from occurring.

1.2.2. *Three levels of pre-positioning*

Setting up an emerging disease control system (in France, a *Système de contrôle des maladies émergentes* (SCME)) involving humans, animals and plants requires pre-positioning at three levels: scientific analysis, primary intervention and secondary intervention. Before going further, it is necessary to point out the idea that any new system of prevention against epidemic emergence must take into account the existing one. This is the case for health monitoring in humans (INVS 2011), animals (ESA 2020) and plants (EOP 2020), and for the structuring of the fight against epidemics, through what was in France the *Établissement de préparation et de réponse aux urgences sanitaires* (EPRUS, Establishment for the Preparation and Response to Health Emergencies). In this regard, it should be noted that this establishment, which is responsible for the important management of FFP2 filtering masks (whose stock was disorganized from 2011 onwards, following criticisms of waste and the shift from a precautionary logic to an accounting logic) (Mercier 2020), was dissolved in 2016 and merged into the *Agence nationale de santé publique* (French National Public Health Agency).

The *"scientific analysis" level* of an SCME implies the collaboration, at the request of the emergency response unit (*Cellule d'intervention sur les émergences* (CNIE), see below) or the Prime Minister's departments, of COR-SCMEs (pre-positioned SCME correspondents) made available by research. These correspondents would be specialized in virology, microbial ecology, parasitology, pathophysiology, toxicology, anatomopathology, biomathematics, informatics, infectiology, epidemiology, law, sociology, psychology and public security (volunteer citizens, who witness the action of the COR-SCMEs, could also be solicited to join the SCME). The team thus constituted could be led, outside of an alert and in the event of an alert, to give advice and act on the basis of a questioning or an injunction from the CNIE, and in connection with a possible, probable or proven emergence.

The *"primary intervention" level* would be handled by a permanent team, the CNIE, stationed in a specific location in a commune near Paris, if we take France as an example. Spearheading preventive control and early biological, statistical and medical analysis of emergencies, as well as intervention actions aimed at deciphering them (conditions and places of emergence, nature of the threat, conditions of its blockage), this team could be composed of 30 to 40 closely-knit people. Thus, the team could include four computer scientists, two computer technicians, four statisticians/modelers, four human and animal pathologists/epidemiologists, two infectious diseases specialists, two biologists, one psychologist, one economist, one librarian, two security guards, two police officers, two nurses, two laboratories, three administrative assistants and three drivers.

This team, in connection with the Prime Minister's services, would propose the passage into a state of pre-alert or alert and would organize interventions in the field during the initial phase of a suspected epidemic process by carrying out investigations and biological samples. Outside of critical phases, the team would contribute the epidemiological and clinical knowledge through the reports it would receive from health professionals and scientists feeding the databases of case notifications, from which the CNIE would build its anti-emergence action. A strange case, instead of corresponding to the "emergence of an emergence", can indeed signify a rare disease, the CNIE being able to contribute in an effective way to a better knowledge of rare diseases in humans and in animals. Moreover, the CNIE, in view of its missions, would have several governmental correspondents, including a principal one at the level of the Prime Minister, and others at the level of the Ministry of Solidarity and Health, the Ministry of the Armed Forces and the Ministry of Agriculture and Food.

The *"secondary intervention" level* would concern a non-permanent departmental intervention team (*Equipe départementale d'intervention* (EDI)), which could be mobilized in an alert situation to analyze the epidemic situation in depth in the affected areas, in order to take over the CNIE interventions. Either this team would be merged with the current regional intervention units (*Cellules d'intervention en région* (Cire)) of the Regional Health Agencies or the EDI would act in coordination with the Cire, while being distinct from them. In terms of each department, the EDI could count on the collaboration of a general practitioner and a public health physician, as well as a veterinarian, an agronomist and a computer technician, depending on the existence of emerging threats. Finally, the idea would be to assemble a maximum of counter-emergency task forces, in order to light effective counter-firewalls to the dissemination of infecting particles or the escape of toxic materials. This could be done using an organization that has points in common with the nuclear risk prevention policy of the *Institut de Radioprotection et de Sûreté Nucléaire* (IRSN, French Institute of Radioprotection and Nuclear Safety) (IRSN 2020), which has levels of intervention that include: alert management; "assessment within the hour"; scenario production; and "multi-level" crisis management.

1.2.3. *Computer tools for anticipation and analysis*

1.2.3.1. *New@Diseases*

The real-time fight against the consequences of epidemiological emergencies in public health, animal health or plant health requires automated and focused monitoring of health dispatches and scientific publications, as tools for understanding the dynamics of diseases. This means monitoring health reports – published in all countries – concerning outbreaks of known diseases and the appearance of possibly new or unexpected clinical expressions in a given area or population.

Of course, in addition to the automated extraction of dispatches, it is necessary to activate networks of correspondents and informants, via, for example, the Pasteur Institutes, foreign universities working in cooperation with French universities and the network of embassies.

In this context, tools for anticipating and analyzing emerging pathologies were developed at INRAE during the 2008–2011 period, including New@Diseases (Figure 1.7), a web application for collecting and analyzing global news on emerging diseases in humans and animals in real time (Barnouin and De Goër 2011).

Connected to news feeds via RSS technology, New@Diseases can collect a variety of news items, which are then analyzed, categorized and stored in a database. The system implements a number of classification criteria, which can vary according to needs.

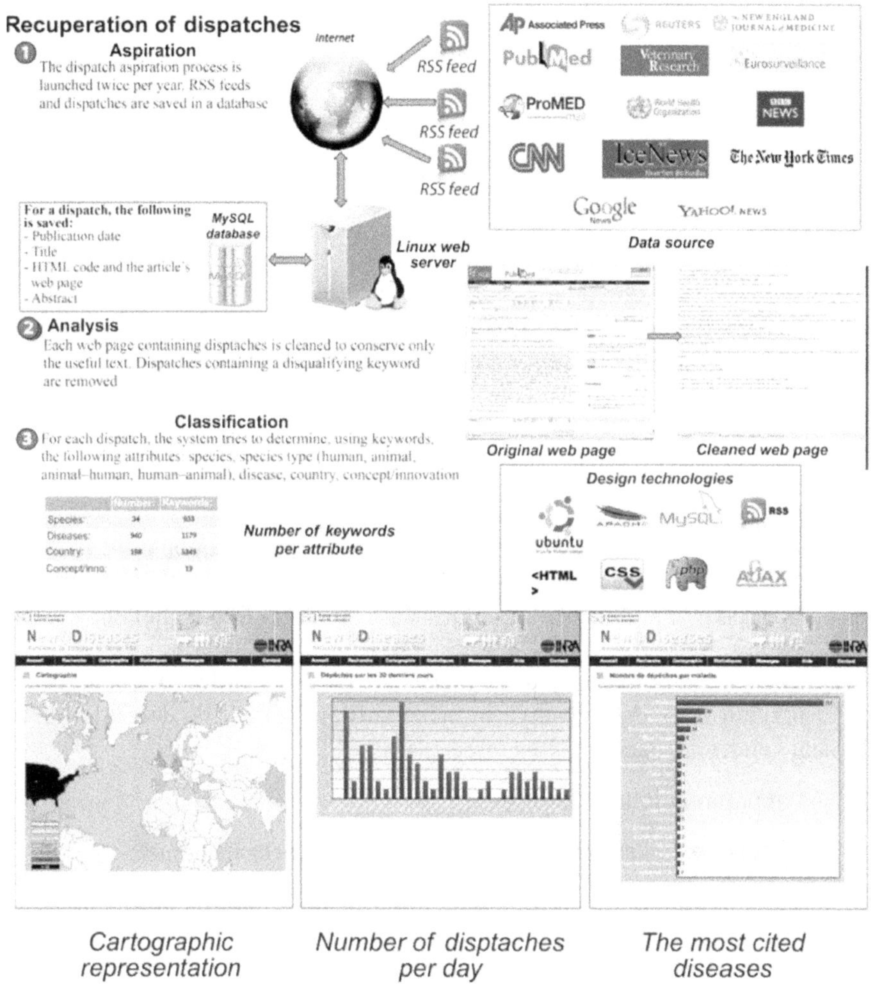
Recuperation of dispatches
1 Aspiration
The dispatch aspiration process is launched twice per year. RSS feeds and dispatches are saved in a database
Internet
RSS feed
RSS feed
RSS feed
For a dispatch, the following is saved:
- Publication date
- Title
- HTML code and the article's web page
- Abstract
MySQL database
Linux web server
Data source
2 Analysis
Each web page containing disptaches is cleaned to conserve only the useful text. Dispatches containing a disqualifying keyword are removed
Original web page
Cleaned web page
Classification
3 For each dispatch, the system tries to determine, using keywords, the following attributes: species, species type (human, animal, animal–human, human–animal), disease, country, concept/innovation
Number of keywords per attribute
Design technologies
Cartographic representation
Number of disptaches per day
The most cited diseases

Figure 1.7. *New@Diseases, a tool for analyzing health dispatches (architecture and graphical output) (source: Bamouin and de Goër 2011). For a color version of this figure, see www.iste.co.uk/salgues/covid.zip*

Within this framework, a website has been developed in order to present, in addition to multi-criteria selection of the dispatches, their statistical information and the geographical location of the information which they carry. It is also possible in the application to generate different RSS feeds allowing the user to be informed in real time. The web pages containing the dispatches processed by New@Diseases (an advanced version of which, called Padi-web or Platform for Automated Extraction of Disease Information from the Web, has since been developed) (Valentin et al. 2020) are cleaned so as to retain only the text useful for the scientific analysis of the information. Dispatches containing a disqualifying keyword are eliminated. For each dispatch, the system then determines the following attributes based on qualifying keywords: species, type of species (human, animal, animal–human, human–animal), disease, country and routine information or information corresponding to a conceptual or technical innovation.

In addition, a website for consulting the results makes it possible to visualize over the current period a possible inflection of the dynamics of the dispatches and the relative importance of their various types.

1.2.3.2. *emergences2*

The emergences2 application, developed in 2008 (Barnouin and Ren 2009) and optimized in collaboration with Sciensano, takes the form of a multilingual site and a database. The application, which can be used to detect and monitor clusters of cases of an emerging disease in animals and humans, has been validated in real-life situations with animals (Behaeghel 2015).

Through emergences2, practitioners are invited to describe online the atypical syndromes they observe in their daily practice. The definition of an atypical syndrome encompasses three cases:

– an apparently unknown disease;

– a disease that is apparently known, but is of a serious nature;

– a known disease not responding to usual treatment or occurring in an unexpected area or time.

A clustering algorithm for similar cases allows a preliminary analysis, through an ascending hierarchical classification method, of reported atypical syndromes and the generation of alerts in case of suspected emergence. All the information gathered can be made available in real time to practitioners, as well as to diagnostic laboratories and research centers, in order to stimulate the exchange of information and the investigation of submitted cases. To perform these tasks, emergences2 includes three types of modules:

– data collection modules;

– modules for making the collected information available;

– automated data analysis modules.

A fourth type of module is reserved for the site's administrator, which allows for management in a multilingual framework. The notification form for clinical cases of emergences2 is the result of a compromise between the minimum time required to enter information (minimized by clear headings and intuitive navigation) and the accuracy of the information collected (Figure 1.8). To allow automated processing of information in the context of a multilingual report, the form reserves a large amount of space for closed fields. In addition to the clinical description, the form includes the precise location of the case and the date of observation of the symptoms. The user is also invited to add photos illustrating the salient aspects of the reported case. A general epidemiological investigation form is integrated into the site, which can be completed in addition to case notification.

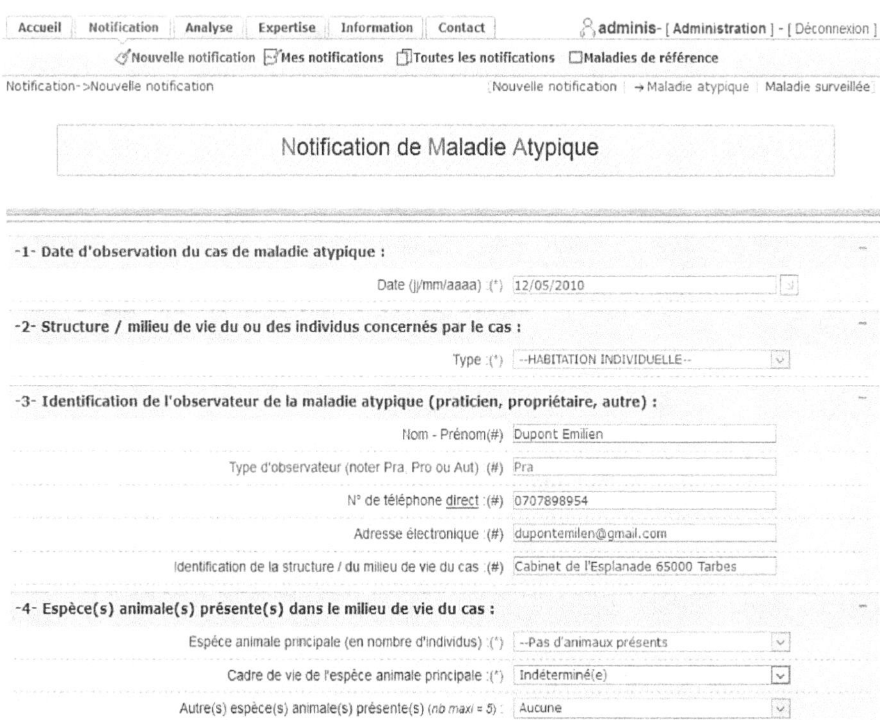

Accueil | Notification | Analyse | Expertise | Information | Contact — adminis- [Administration] - [Déconnexion]

Nouvelle notification | Mes notifications | Toutes les notifications | Maladies de référence

Notification->Nouvelle notification — Nouvelle notification | → Maladie atypique | Maladie surveillée

Notification de Maladie Atypique

-1- Date d'observation du cas de maladie atypique :

Date (jj/mm/aaaa) :(*) 12/05/2010

-2- Structure / milieu de vie du ou des individus concernés par le cas :

Type :(*) --HABITATION INDIVIDUELLE--

-3- Identification de l'observateur de la maladie atypique (praticien, propriétaire, autre) :

Nom - Prénom(#) Dupont Emilien

Type d'observateur (noter Pra, Pro ou Aut) (#) Pra

N° de téléphone direct :(#) 0707898954

Adresse électronique :(#) dupontemilen@gmail.com

Identification de la structure / du milieu de vie du cas :(#) Cabinet de l'Esplanade 65000 Tarbes

-4- Espèce(s) animale(s) présente(s) dans le milieu de vie du cas :

Espèce animale principale (en nombre d'individus) :(*) --Pas d'animaux présents

Cadre de vie de l'espèce animale principale :(*) Indéterminé(e)

Autre(s) espèce(s) animale(s) présente(s) (nb maxi = 5) : Aucune

Figure 1.8. *Partial view of the notification form for an atypical syndrome in the emergences2 application (source: J. Barnouin)*

In addition to identifying and viewing their own notifications, the emergences2 application allows users to access notifications from other practitioners. For these notifications, the data allowing the univocal identification of the reporter is obviously hidden. In this way, the user can view all the notifications made in a geographical area over the last few months (Figure 1.9). Finally, in order to provide elements of reflection on a specific case of interest, emergences2 allows users to visualize the most similar notifications to this case. The calculation of similarity between notifications is based on the clinical picture and the type of patient affected, as well as the spatial and temporal proximity of the cases. One of the challenges of a real-time detection system is the efficient use of the data to generate an early warning of an outbreak.

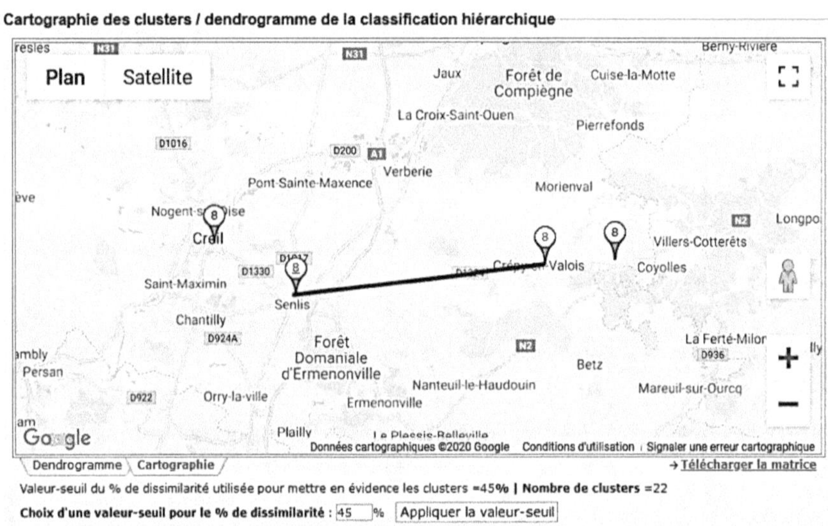

Figure 1.9. *Mapping module of the emergences2 application. Example of a visualization of a cluster of four cases of an atypical syndrome attributable to Covid-19 and occurring in France in the Oise department (the two initial cases of cluster no. 8 are linked by a dark line, the number of the first case being underlined) (source: J. Barnouin, based on Google Maps, cartographic data © 2020 Google). For a color version of this figure, see www.iste.co.uk/salgues/covid.zip*

To allow automated analysis of the information, emergences2 uses an unsupervised aggregation method for notifications. Aggregation (or clustering) is a process for grouping data into homogeneous groups (or clusters), which implies that objects in the same group have a high similarity to each other and are conversely very different from objects in other groups (Han and Kamber 2006) (Figure 1.10). Initially, each object is placed in its own group. The groups are then merged based on a similarity index into larger groups, until only one group remains or an imposed condition is met (e.g. that a minimum degree of similarity between two groups is reached) to merge them. The so-called "unsupervised" approach makes it possible to group notifications without knowing a priori the number of existing categories or their characteristics. The unsupervised approach applies very well to the detection of emerging diseases whose clinical and epidemiological characteristics are not necessarily known a priori. As for alerting the system – through atypical cases suspected of reflecting an emergence – this must, of course, be done by all the medical and health structures capable of diagnosing a suspected case, the contributions of practitioners and hospital practitioners being decisive at this level via traditional practices, structures such as SOS Médecins, hospital emergency departments and clinics.

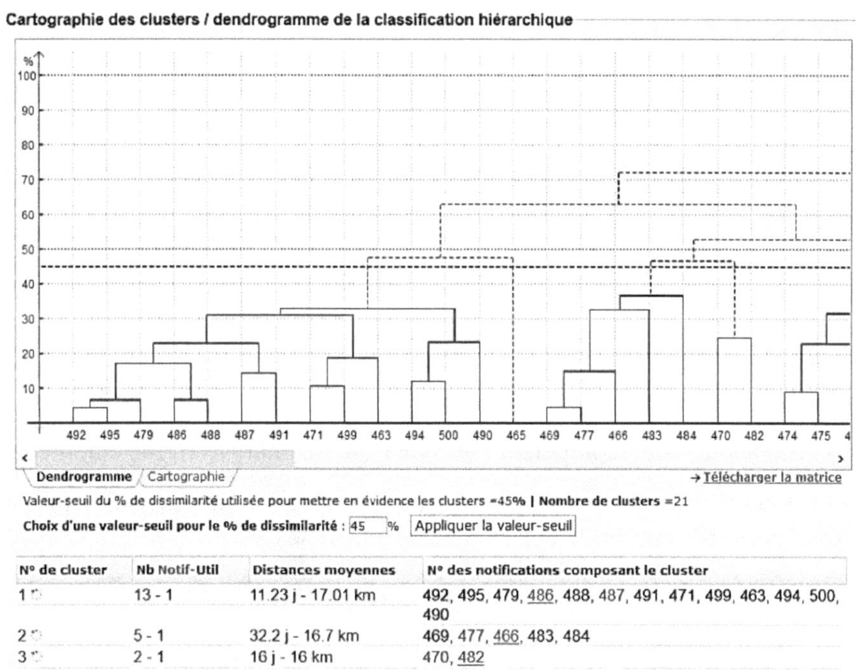

Figure 1.10. *Dendrogram of the hierarchical classification of the emergences2 application allowing the detection and analysis of clusters (source: J. Barnouin). For a color version of this figure, see www.iste.co.uk/salgues/covid.zip*

1.3. Health rules and scientific lines of thought and action

In addition to the pre-positioning of the epidemic control system, for which the best organization must be found, the tools for analyzing the emergence that have just been presented can be optimized through predictive modeling, propagation scenarios and the study of the consequences of anti-epidemic measures. The fight against emergence also requires the definition of decision rules, some of which were presented in the first part of the discussion. A set of supplies (stocks of FFP2 filtering masks) and quarantine locations – with automatic temperature control – a policy of early detection of case-contacts and the adoption of rules applicable to personnel working in the aeronautical industry or monitoring borders also seem to be defined in the alert phase.

As for public research, it should be prepositioned in a sustainable manner on the issue of emerging risks, based on questions such as deciphering the conditions of "appearance" and "disappearance" of viruses; the immune response of a sample of animal species to viruses that are potentially deleterious to humans; the factors that modulate the inflammatory response (over- or under-reaction) to viral infections, and the questions raised in this respect by "Western seniors", with reference to Covid-19; rapid screening and tracing techniques; methods for accelerated development of vaccines (see on this point Chapter 2); virus surveillance (and diagnosis in medical practice); and the development of innovative tools for controlling emerging epidemics, which is one of the issues specifically addressed in this chapter.

Here are the main lines of thought to be implemented in order to control emerging diseases, taken from the *Émergences 2006* symposium organized by INRAE (Sache and Barnouin 2006):

1) train and assign competent observers for the analysis of the emergence;

2) strengthen surveillance by setting up specific interdisciplinary and inter-agency mechanisms devoted to emerging diseases;

3) observe the evolution of agricultural, agro-industrial and consumer practices that may be linked to the emergence;

4) initiate early detection of pathological atypia through operational training systems operating in real time;

5) systematically collect standardized epidemiological information during – and in anticipation of – emergencies;

6) develop automated analytical methods for unbiased detection to characterize emerging pathologies;

7) develop statistical and modeling methods adapted to the issue of epidemiological emergence;

8) broaden the issue of emergence from infectious diseases;

9) clarify the central issue of crossing the species barrier by strengthening the work on the epidemiological conditions of this crossing;

10) formalize structural links (e.g. through the creation of joint research teams) between plant health, animal health and human health specialists;

11) empower all actors involved in the detection and analysis of emerging diseases to ensure their active and continuous participation;

12) bring scientific research and field practices closer together in the area of emergence by establishing permanent links between these two circles;

13) optimize international cooperation and refine global information systems on emerging diseases;

14) draw up a typology and study the cyclicity of past emergences, as a tool for future reflection;

15) conceptualize emergence through biological deciphering and modeling of "model pathosystems" determined through an interdisciplinary scientific consensus.

It remains to be seen why the proposals for action that have just been formulated have not been implemented, even though they appear to be consistent with a better understanding of epidemiological emergencies. Why did we miss them? No doubt because "we" have shown an excess of conservatism, a good pinch of humdrum, a bit of arrogance and a difficulty in really welcoming health and safety innovation. This is particularly true of administrations, which can sometimes administer with the idea of consolidating their position and guaranteeing their peace in the present, rather than preparing for the future and exposing themselves, and because "we" do not give enough space to prevention, which is costly in the short term, restrictive and uninspiring in its content. Basically, it can be said that there is a kind of global inefficiency in the large administered states in dealing reactively with the non-standard and the unforeseen and questioning their procedures and practices, in order to take the calculated risks that are necessary, in unforeseen situations. Thus, the development of an advanced form of state-strategist, both a guarantor of the general interest and perfectly capable of initiative and agility, in the manner of companies, is one of the major challenges that all democratic societies urgently face, through the Covid-19 pandemic crisis.

Other organizational factors may have contributed to the unpreparedness to the crisis, such as the fact that scientific structures in France do not have procedures for examining the opportunity to save strategic programs following a redeployment of resources or the end of the career of certain researchers. For example, the development of emergences2 was prematurely halted in 2011–2012, even though this application was a pioneer. Furthermore, to take another significant example, a French team of very high-level researchers – working at INRAE on animal coronaviruses and led by Hubert Laude – was reoriented in 1997, by authority and to the great displeasure of the researchers, towards the study of prion diseases (Larousserie 2020).

1.4. Geographical distribution of Covid-19 cases and differences in population susceptibility to SARS-CoV-2 infection

1.4.1. *Analyzing the geography of the epidemic to better understand it*

"Without allowing ourselves to be won over by catastrophist theories, such as those featuring the destructive action of a supervirus gaining perfect knowledge of our genome" (Barnouin 2020), will we have to act more circumspectly, now that the Covid-19 crisis is impacting us, to better protect ourselves in the future from the risks of viral emergence? In this perspective and in order to respond to the challenges of SARS-CoV-2, will we now have to develop collaborative constructions involving scientists, practitioners, decision-makers and societal actors in the long term, in order to move towards "all responsible and all useful" societies and not "permanent individual whining"? One of the challenges to be met in this perspective is to analyze the geography of Covid-19 in order to better understand the lifestyle habits that promote or hinder the spread of SARS-CoV-2 to populations.

In addition to the factors that led to the emergence of the "new SARS", we will also have to uncover the reasons for the large differences in the severity of the epidemic between countries (Figure 1.11). Thus, on July 15, 2020, for example, there were twice as many deaths in France as in India, a proportion that was reversed in January 2021, with a mortality rate that was nevertheless 10 times higher in France, a developed country, than in India, which is one of the less prosperous countries; and to compare two prosperous countries, there were 10 times more cases in France than in Japan (127 million inhabitants) on April 21 (and 18 times more in France in January 2021). As for South Africa, a country with a similar population size to France, by the end of April it had experienced 34 times fewer cases than France. Here again, although the number of cases changed significantly following the spring period (e.g. it increased significantly in India), the changes observed at the end of the summer do not really call into question the major findings of the end of April, even though we can question the exhaustiveness of the registration of cases, which differs between countries according to organizational, technical, religious and political factors. For example, we have received unofficial information from North Africa, which suggests that deaths attributed to SARS-CoV-2 in that region of the world may have been underestimated.

1.4.2. *Covid-19 in the world*

At this stage of the epidemic – and given our still-frustrated knowledge of SARS-CoV-2 – it is not easy to comment on the map in Figure 1.11. Nevertheless, it seems to show a strong susceptibility, direct (genetic?) or indirect (linked to international contacts?), to Covid-19 of prosperous Western European populations in their matrix states and in states (United States, Canada, Australia, New Zealand) with predominantly European populations. If we look at the map of the areas that have been little affected by the pandemic and those that have been heavily affected, differences in temperature and humidity could help explain the differences in the extent of the epidemic between countries. Indeed, high temperatures (and high levels of air humidity) slow down the pathogenicity and/or transmissibility of the coronavirus and would also be favorable to the functioning of immune defenses, as is suspected for influenza (Fuhrmann 2010).

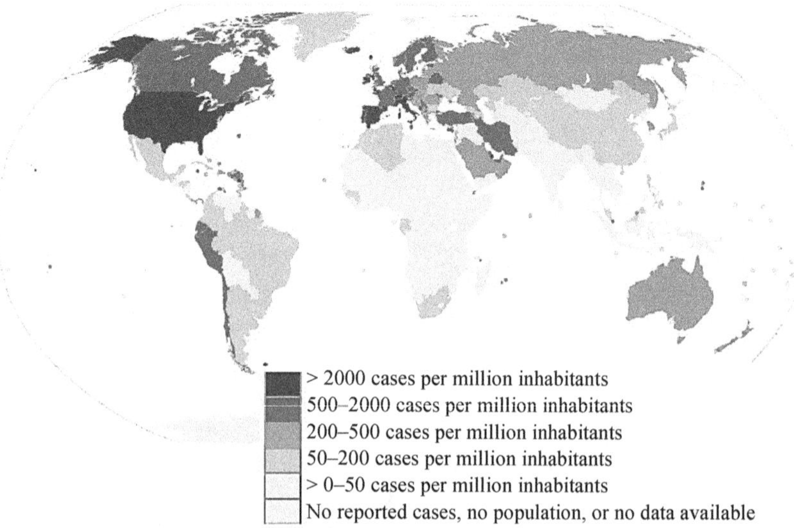

Figure 1.11. *Number of Covid-19 cases per country and per million inhabitants on April 21, 2020 (source: Raphaël Dunant 2020). For a color version of this figure, see www.iste.co.uk/salgues/covid.zip*

In this regard, we note that Africa, the hottest (Barnouin 2020) and least prosperous continent, is the least affected by Covid-19 (Figure 1.12), with 1,200 deaths as of April 21, 2020, compared to 106,000 in Europe on that date (a trend that has not changed since). This is despite the fact that the African continent is home to 1.3 billion people and that the World Health Organization (WHO) predicted a "Covid-19-related health catastrophe, if Africa does not wake up" (Chapuis 2020). What is "Africa's secret", if it persists (the response is yes), and the statistics published by African countries reflect the reality of the epidemic? A very young population? Natural or cross-immunity through other diseases, especially parasitic? High average temperatures? In terms of climate, northern Italy, which is colder (and more economically active) than its southern part, has more cases of Covid-19 than the latter (Figure 1.13). For example, Lazio, the south-central region with the capital city of Rome (mean annual temperature: 17.6°C), had 5,895 Covid-19 cases as of April 21, 2020, compared to 67,931 cases observed in Milan (mean annual temperature: 13°C), that is, 150 cases per 100,000 inhabitants in Lazio compared to 720 in Lombardy. The climatic hypothesis should therefore be considered with regard to the Covid-19 risk, as well as the major epidemic factors, which are the early appearance of the disease in a region (Lombardy and Veneto in Italy) and the virulence and contagiousness of the viral variants in circulation.

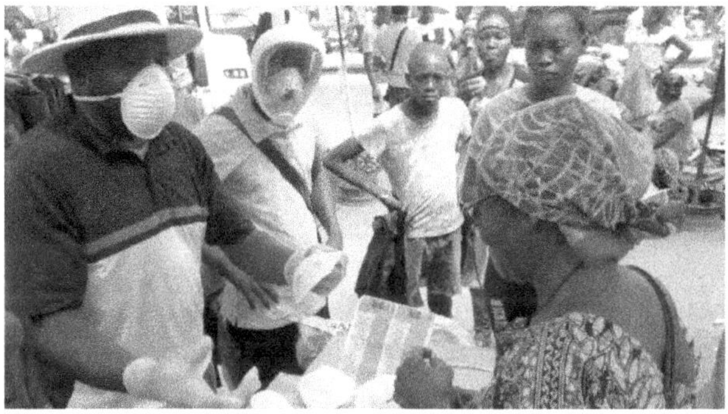

Figure 1.12. *Mask vendor in Brazzaville, Republic of Congo, during the Covid-19 pandemic (source: VOA/Arsène Séverin 2020)*

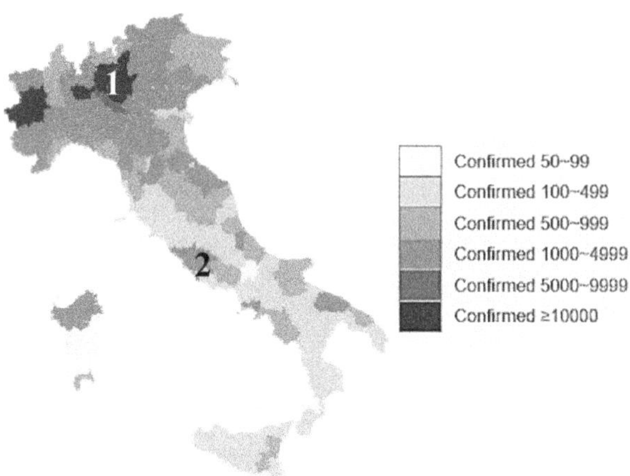

Figure 1.13. *Number of Covid-19 cases in Italy by region as of February 27, 2020. Legend: 1 = Lombardy; 2 = Lazio (source: Facquis 2020). For a color version of this figure, see www.iste.co.uk/salgues/covid.zip*

As for the potentially seasonal nature of Covid-19 (Amani et al. 2020), whose epidemic pattern appears to be quite classical up to now, although unprecedented in its universality, it could be translated, via the evolution of strains and the increase in temperature and sunshine (whose partially deleterious effect on the virus has been reported (Amani et al. 2020; Baker et al. 2020; Riddell et al. 2020; Wu et al. 2020b)) into:

1) the decline, in Europe, of the most serious consequences of the epidemic, with a very sharp drop in mortality at the end of spring 2020, and a spectacular rebound from September–October onwards attributable to a reduction in sanitary precautions and the increased contagiousness of the virus (Figure 1.14); the impact of this rebound in terms of mortality appeared both very significant and relatively moderate, in relation to the evolution of the ratio "number of new deaths divided by the number of new cases per day", which was 20 times lower in mid-October than it had been up to then on average (however, "what a case is" has evolved with the progression of testing, the October cases concerning mainly cases with few or no symptoms which would have been only slightly detectable in April, given the absence of mass screening at that date);

2) a sharp increase in cases in the southern hemisphere, following the onset of the southern winter; this increase was nevertheless followed by a decline in cases from mid-September onwards, particularly in Australia.

Apart from climatic and viral evolution parameters, the factors to be tested to explain the differences in national incidences of Covid-19 appear to be:

– the virulence dynamics of the strains, which are difficult to evaluate;

– travel from epidemic areas (France was particularly affected by the contamination from China, as this country alone accounts for 55% of Chinese tourists visiting Europe);

– population density;

– the quality of social distancing, both natural and regulated;

– the distribution of age groups;

– the lifestyle of the elderly;

– the incidences of diabetes, hypertension and obesity;

– geographical isolation (Figure 1.15);

– the earliness of the lockdown and screening process.

Thus, European countries with high-quality health structures, but ultimately impacted by the epidemic, may have, in addition to unfavorable genetic factors (Hadjadj et al. 2020), combined provirus factors such as:

– circulation of virulent variants;

– numerous arrivals of people from outbreaks;

– a high proportion of senior citizens (more than 20% of Europeans are over 65, compared to less than 4% of Africans and nearly 7% of Indians);

– social habits involving a high density of contacts and relative indiscipline with regard to health instructions;

– insufficiently early and large-scale lockdown and screening.

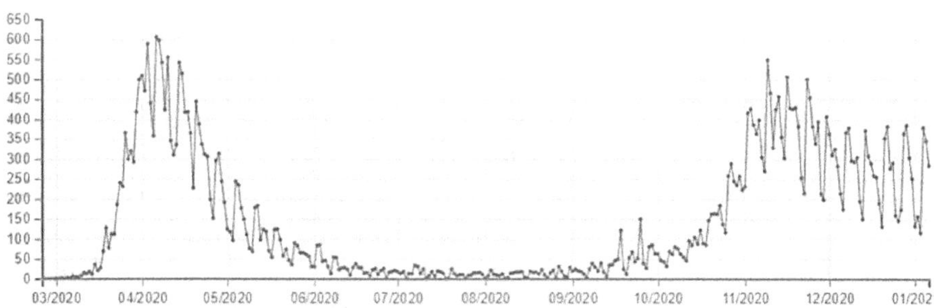

Figure 1.14. *Daily deaths attributed to Covid-19 in hospitals in France from March 2020 to January 2021 (source: Wikipedia 2021)*

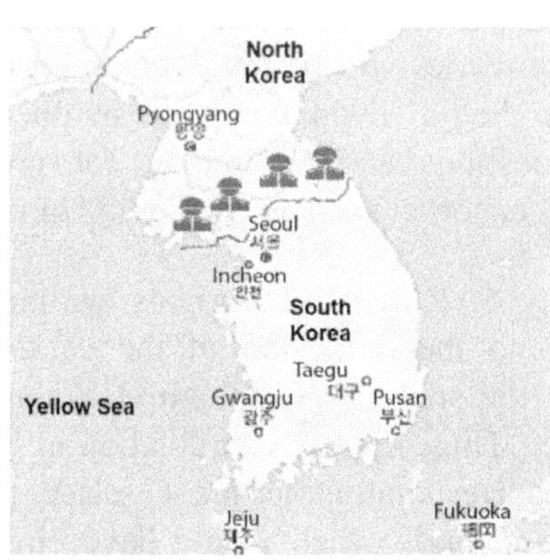

Figure 1.15. *South Korea, an example of geographical isolation (and anti-epidemic organization): the sea on three sides and a militarized border in the north (source: J. Barnouin and Google Maps 2020)*

1.4.3. *Possible explanations for differences in population susceptibility to SARS-CoV-2*

One possible explanation for the differences in sensitivity of populations to SARS-CoV-2 is that for a virus to infect a cell, it must attach itself, via a protein in its envelope, to a protein (a *receptor*) located on the cell membrane. Thus, it is ACE2 (Angiotensin-Converting Enzyme 2) which, together with the serine protease TMPRSS2 (Transmembrane Serine Protease 2) (Hoffmann 2020), is thought to play the role of a gateway for SARS-CoV-2, while at the same time participating in the regulation of arterial pressure (which would explain the sensitivity of diabetics and hypertensives to Covid-19, whose arterial pressure is already poorly regulated) (Alifano et al. 2020). For example, studies conducted in an animal model have shown a positive correlation between the level of expression of ACE2 and the risk of developing Covid-19 (Société française de pharmacologie et de thérapeutique 2020), and in humans, a relationship has been observed between this risk, certain variants of ACE2 and their interactions with viral spike proteins (Hussain et al. 2020). Anything that could block the expression of the virus via ACE2 should therefore be at the heart of research on SARS-CoV-2. Drug candidates are being studied, such as hrsACE2, which would almost completely inhibit the viral load (Monteil et al. 2020). However, blocking the virus via ACE2 could have negative consequences on the regulation of blood pressure, except perhaps in the case of treatment limited in time. Finally, ACE2 receptors, which have higher circulating concentrations in men than in women, are thought to be one explanation for the higher risk of Covid-19 in men (Sama et al. 2020). Nevertheless, new discoveries will be made regarding the interaction of the virus with the human body, given the large number of scientific teams working on these questions and federating, for greater efficiency, via international research consortia, such as the Covid Human Genetic Effort[2].

The distribution of SARS-CoV-2 variants within populations is still relatively unknown (and the definition of the variant and strain is still unclear), even though the study by Gámbaro et al. in 2020 provides some insight into the subject. Thus, the early circulation in France of a variant of undetermined origin corresponding to the G clade (a clade includes an ancestor and its descendants), which would have circulated mainly at the beginning of the epidemic, has been pointed out. The different countries

2 Covid Human Genetic Effort website: https://www.covidhge.com.

could therefore have been affected by more or less pathogenic clades, with one study revealing that some variants were 270 times more virulent than others (Yao et al. 2020), with the strains circulating in Europe ("exported" to New York) being the most pathogenic (Korber et al. 2020), with a greater number of mutations in Europe than elsewhere and a total number of mutations of the order of perhaps 10 (Islam et al. 2020). Although this number may differ according to the authors, the mutations detected generate copies of the original virus that are sufficiently close to the latter for it to be reasonable to think that the pathogenic action of all the strains in circulation can be countered by the action of a standard vaccine (Goffard 2020). The problem of viral variations, with its numerous developments (including English, South African, Brazilian, Californian, Lambda, Mu, Delta and Omicron strains, the latter being predominant in October 2021) (California Department of Public Health, 2021) and the unknowns that remain, could possibly be studied in an original way in Iceland, a country that is very little affected by Covid-19 (29 deaths at the end of January 2021) and genetically homogeneous and geographically isolated. Thus, DeCODE Genetics, an Iceland-based company (Offord 2017) specializing in genome analysis, is working to investigate "the burning question" of factors related to the low level of contamination of "the land of ice" by SARS-CoV-2 (nevertheless, this initial low level is no longer really relevant, as 13,500 cases were registered in the country in October 2021).

1.5. Conclusion: challenging, preparing, uniting

1.5.1. *A manageable crisis*

While no one appears "especially guilty" of the occurrence of the Covid-19 crisis, it is highly unfortunate that real-time epidemic threat analysis systems, whose annual cost can be estimated at 1/10,000th the cost of the epidemic, were not used to contain SARS-CoV-2. Overall, the coronavirus crisis was controllable, if not preventable, given the existence of:

1) at the national level:

- pre-positioned systems for early detection and decryption of epidemics,

- strict sanitary rules for the various factors in the fight against the epidemic, including early and detailed containment and control of sources of contamination,

- sufficient stocks of hygiene materials (masks, disinfectants);

2) at the international level:

- coordination of national early detection systems and the existence of an international scientific body temporarily available for the coordinated development of screening tests and therapeutic and vaccine trials,

- early screening of international travelers.

However, as such precautions were not taken for the most part, egos, conservatism and the lack of a preventive spirit led, in a large number of countries including France, to decisions being taken at the beginning of the epidemic that were ill-adapted to the dynamics and seriousness of the crisis; this is in contrast to what happened in certain countries, notably Taiwan and South Korea, as well as in China, which succeeded in containing the epidemic relatively well, even though it was the "birthplace" of the disease.

As for South Korea, which has been very little affected by Covid-19, only 2,850 deaths due to SARS-CoV-2 were reported in this country of 52 million inhabitants until October 2021, and for good reason:

> According to the French ambassador in Seoul, one of the country's assets was the previous existence of a real "staff structure" activated at the time of the crisis, with a pre-established escalation plan. South Korea is a military model based on intelligence, analysis, command and control. It is an organization, more than an accumulation of resources, that has proven to be effective in this country (Magal 2020).

Moreover, the Covid-19 crisis has shown the lack of independence of many nations, including France, with respect to the production of essential drugs (Gleize 2020) and health materials, and has been the scene of endless controversy over the effectiveness of anti-SRAS-CoV-2 control measures and treatments, with everyone occasionally becoming a doctor, infectious disease specialist, epidemiologist or vaccinologist. Regarding treatment, it seems that anti-corona therapy must, in addition to neutralizing the virus (Wang et al. 2020), control its ability to reach the brain via the olfactory bulb (Pouga 2020) and trigger a "cytokine storm" (Émilie et al. 2020; Zhou et al. 2020), that is, generate an "overreaction of the organism", which has led to many deaths from respiratory distress. To succeed, it is necessary to consider in therapeutic research protocols, as many scientific teams are now doing, all the effectors of inflammation (cytokines, complement system, white blood cells), both in fragile versus resistant individuals and animal models (Peffault de Latour et al. 2020; Schulte-Schrepping et al. 2020).

To date, synthetic corticosteroids, including dexamethasone (Johnson and Vimetz 2020), appear to be the most successful in treating hyperinflammatory Covid patients, as well as molnupiravir, an antiviral which appears to contain the replication of SARS-CoV-2 and lower the risk of death by 50%, but whose price is particularly high. Ongoing research will also make it possible to broaden therapeutics, in particular through the identification of genetic flaws used by the virus to multiply, including type 1 interferon deficiencies (Hadjadj et al. 2020). Thus, these molecules could be used to combat the virus by injection or inhalation (Bélier 2020). In addition, testing thousands of drugs – already known and used in diseases other than Covid-19 – for their ability to annihilate SARS-CoV-2, is a promising research method that would allow the identification of a drug candidate via the Institut Pasteur de Lille (France) (Lemke 2020). Injecting a cocktail of artificial antibodies that bind to the surface of SARS-CoV-2 and prevent it from attaching to the cells through which the virus attempts to multiply is another therapeutic avenue (Cavicchioli 2020). Finally, the fact that prior infection with a common cold coronavirus appears to reduce the severity of Covid-19 disease, including in particular the risk of admission to intensive care, is a finding that could be usefully exploited in the fight against pandemic coronavirus (Sagar 2020).

1.5.2. *A crisis without a written end*

The continuation – and end – of the pandemic will depend on:

– the genetic evolution of the virus and the direction of this possible evolution, in terms of pathogenicity and contagiousness;

– the appropriateness of – and degree of compliance by the population with – the control measures;

– the speed of development of accessible treatments, and above all of effective vaccines against SARS-CoV-2 (whose distribution began from the end of 2020 to the beginning of 2021 in the form of classic or messenger RNA-based vaccines, and which should be allowed to benefit all the nations of the world as soon as possible, for the sake of justice and the effectiveness of the anti-pandemic fight);

– international cooperation, in terms of providing vaccines to vulnerable populations and fighting extreme poverty (Hiault 2020);

– the quality of acquired immunity following the circulation of SARS-CoV-2 in populations and a first infection.

With respect to this last listed parameter, the number of reported cases of reinfection appears to be very low. Of the five initial cases reported (in Hong Kong, Belgium, Ecuador, the Netherlands and the United States) between the beginning of the epidemic and October 2020, the second infection was more severe than the first in two cases, and less severe in the other three, and in the American case of reinfection, for which an extensive investigation was conducted, genetic analysis showed that the two successive infections were caused by two different strains of SARS-CoV-2, which may be reassuring (Tillett et al. 2020). Nevertheless, according to Akiko Iwasaki:

> reinfection cases tell us that we cannot rely on immunity acquired by natural infection to confer herd immunity; not only is this strategy lethal for many, but also it is not effective. Herd immunity requires safe and effective vaccines and robust vaccination implementation (Iwasaki 2020).

The actual end of the Covid-19 pandemic is almost impossible to predict. Apart from the influences on SARS-CoV-2 activity of herd immunity, the genetic evolution of the virus, climatic parameters, the effectiveness of disease control and the widespread availability of vaccines and treatments, the factors behind the "disappearance" of viruses are not known. For example, the sudden end of the A/H1N1 pandemics in 2009, or SARS-CoV in 2003, cannot be explained. Consequently, we can only predict a bright future for work in viral ecology (O'Malley 2016) and the multifactorial study of virus–genetic environment interactions at the basis of viral circulations.

1.5.3. *A crisis alien to our societal software*

Finally, the difficulty in managing the Covid-19 crisis does not seem unrelated to the fact that this type of event is not (any more) part of the software of a large number of the planet's inhabitants. Indeed, a certain number of *sapiens* in affluent countries are now too busy consuming and navigating in virtual universes, cut off from the balance of nature – and more libertarians than citizens – to accept that a virus should upset their appetites, interfere with their plans and make them obey orders "from above". Moreover, national decision-makers, grappling with the partly contradictory imperatives of public health and economic health, and scrutinized 24 hours a day by the media and social networks (prone to dramatize the slightest hitch), have a hard time enacting anti-epidemic measures that are seen as being in the general interest, which is now competing not only with the disparate sum of particular interests but also with the uncontrollable and fluctuating palette of individual desires. In this climate of mistrust and cookie-cutter actions, which creates – with difficulty –solid common sense, it is not surprising that a French artist could declare in September 2020, rebelling against the mask and barrier gestures:

> Live hard, get sick, go to restaurants, yell at the cops, contradict your bosses and the cowardly government directives. We must live now, even if it means dying [our elderly need tenderness more than our precautions]. We must stop stopping. We live. We love. We have fever. We move forward. We pull out of the gray area. It's not the color of our hearts.

Yes, the crisis has been difficult to live through. Yes, it has locked us in. Yes, it has blurred the future. Yes, it has been strange to phone a distant country and find that everywhere we have experienced the same uncertainties, the same symptoms, the same suffering and the same limitations. The crisis that has worried us – and is worrying us – is a bit like suffering a new kind of world war, having to fight an invisible, unpredictable and well-armed aggressor. From now on, perhaps we will be a little more united, perhaps we will relativize our small problems more easily, because of the common and impactful ordeal that we had to face?

Before closing the deciphering, let us once again think of the victims of the pandemic, too often reduced to statistical objects by media announcements. Let us thank with immense gratitude all those who have contributed to the fight against the epidemic through their qualities as lovers, leaders, workers and citizens, and above all as caregivers. Finally, let us be guided by the words of the Italian writer Paolo Giordano, in the conclusion of his book *Contagions*:

> We can tell ourselves that Covid-19 is an isolated accident, a disgrace or a plague, crying that it is all their fault. There is nothing to stop us. Or we can work to make sense of the

contagion. Make better use of that time, use it to ponder what normality prevents us from pondering: how we got here, how we would like to get on with our lives. Count the days. Apply our hearts to wisdom. Not to allow all this suffering to pass in vain (Giordano 2020).

1.6. References

Abat, C., Chaudet, H., Rolain, J.-M., Colson, P., Raoult, D. (2016). Traditional and syndromic surveillance of infectious diseases and pathogens. *International Journal of Infectious Diseases*, 48, 22–28.

Alifano, M., Alifano, P., Forgez, P., Iannelli, A. (2020). Renin-angiotensin system at the heart of Covid-19 pandemic. *Biochimie*, 174, 30–33.

Amani, A., Malak, A., Malak, K., Ghina, H., Hadi, Y.M., Hassan, Z. (2020). Seasonality of respiratory viral infections: Will Covid-19 follow suit? *Frontiers in Public Health*, 8, 576. doi=10.3389/fpubh.2020.567184.

Bacqué, R. and Pedroletti, B. (2020). Coronavirus: Les laboratoires de Wuhan, épicentres de la rumeur. *Le Monde*, 25 April.

Baker, R.E., Yang, W., Vecchi, G.A., Metcalf, C.J.E., Grenfell, B.T. (2020). Susceptible supply limits the role of climate in the early SARS-CoV-2 pandemic. *Science*, 369(6501), 315–319.

Barnouin, J. (2009). Survey and cluster potential emerging diseases: An attempt at answer through emergences2. *9th Annual Symposium on Zoonotic and Communicable Diseases*, Vancouver [Online]. Available at: https://www.researchgate.net/publication/285592716_Survey_and_cluster_potential_emerging_diseases_an_attempt_at_answer_through_emergences2_Towards_a_follow-up_in_real-time_of_the_evolution_of_disease_pattern_among_animal_species.

Barnouin, J. (2012). Les menaces épidémiologiques de nature zoonotique et la mise en place de nouveaux concepts de surveillance. In *Les maladies émergentes et le franchissement des barrières d'espèces*, Hervé, C., Hintermeyer, P., Rozenberg, J.J. (eds). De Boeck, Louvain-la-Neuve.

Barnouin, J. (2020). *The World's Construction Mechanism: Trajectories, Imbalances and the Future of Societies*. ISTE Ltd, London, and Wiley, New York.

Barnouin, J. and De Goër, J. (2011). New@Diseases, un outil de veille stratégique en temps réel sur les maladies émergentes. *Journées d'Animation Scientifique du département de santé animale de l'INRA*. Fréjus.

Barnouin, J. and Ren, L. (2009). Documentation du système d'information épidémiologique émergences2. Unité de Recherche d'Épidémiologie Animale INRA, Clermont-Ferrand [Online]. Available at: https://www.researchgate.net/publication/275973716_Epidemiological_Information_System_emergences2_guidelines_Systeme_d'Information_Epidemiologique_emergences2_documentation.

Barnouin, J. and Sache, I. (2010). *Épidémiologie des maladies émergentes chez le Végétal, l'Animal et l'Homme*. Quae, Versailles.

Barnouin, J. and Vourc'h, G. (2004). Les maladies émergentes: Un défi pour le développement durable des productions animales. *INRA Productions Animales*, 17(5), 355–363.

Barnouin, J., Verdura Barrios, T., Chassagne, M., Pérez Cristiá, R., Arnaud, J., Fleites Mestre, P., Esther Montoya, M., Favier, A. (2001). Nutritional and food protection against epidemic emerging neuropathy. Epidemiological findings in the unique disease-free urban area of Cuba. *International Journal of Vitamin and Nutrition Research*, 71(5), 274–285.

Behaeghel, I., Veldhuis, A., Ren, L., Méroc, E., Koenen, F., Kerkhofs, P., Van der Stede, Y., Barnouin, J., Dispas, M. (2015). Evaluation of a hierarchical ascendant clustering process implemented in a veterinary syndromic surveillance system. *Preventive Veterinary Medicine*, 120(2), 141–151.

Bélier, A. (2020). Un traitement contre la Covid-19 jugé prometteur au Royaume-Uni. *Sud-Ouest*, 25 January.

BFM TV (2020). Coronavirus: Des premiers cas en Outre-mer, à Saint-Martin et St-Barth. *BFM TV*, 1 March.

Bouhaut, F. and Rosique, A. (2020). Coronavirus: Un troisième patient hospitalisé à Lyon, 38 cas confirmés en France. *BFM TV*, 27 February.

California Departement of Public Health (2021). COVID-19 variant first found in other countries and states now seen more frequently in California. L452R Variant is linked to multiple outbreaks in Santa Clara county and being studied by California genomic sequencing experts [Online]. Available at: https://www.cdph.ca.gov/Programs/OPA/Pages/NR21-020.aspx.

Cao, Y., Li, L., Feng, Z., Wan, S., Huang, P., Sun, X., Wen, F., Huang, X., Ning, G., Wang, W. (2020). Comparative genetic analysis of the novel coronavirus (2019-nCoV/SARS-CoV-2) receptor ACE2 in different populations. *Cell Discovery*, 6(11) [Online]. Available at: https://doi.org/10.1038/s41421-020-0147-1.

Castéra, I. (2020). Patient bordelais contaminé par le Covid-19: J'ai d'abord voulu protéger les miens. *Sud-Ouest*, 25 January.

Cavicchioli, L. (2020). L'espoir des anticorps antiviraux dans la lutte contre le Covid-19. *The Conversation*, 3 August.

Chapuis, E. (2020). Coronavirus: L'Afrique appelée par l'OMS à se préparer au pire et dès aujourd'hui. *Sciences et Avenir*, 20 March.

Chubb (2019). Baromètre des risques émergents, édition 2018 [Online]. Available at: https://www.chubb.com/fr-fr/_assets/documents/20190129_chubb_risques-emergents_vfinale.pdf.

Coq-Chodorge, C. (2020). Les hôpitaux français touchés par le coronavirus. *Mediapart*, 28 February.

Costentin, P. and Genton, P. (2020). Coronavirus: Ce que l'on sait sur le rassemblement religieux à Mulhouse d'où viennent de nombreuses maladies. *France-Bleu Haut-Rhin*, 5 March.

Courrier Picard (2020a). Coronavirus: L'armée française au défi de continuer ses missions. *Courrier Picard*, 11 March.

Courrier Picard (2020b). Coronavirus: Les Ehpad de Crépy en première ligne. *Courrier Picard*, 10 March.

Cristiani, J. (2020). Coronavirus: Soigné au remdesivir, le patient de Bordeaux, qui venait de Wuhan, est tiré d'affaire. *La Tribune*, 14 February.

Dargnies, G. (2020). Je criais à Jésus de secourir ma voisine de chambre, raconte une rescapée du coronavirus. *Famille Chrétienne*, 17 March.

De Filippis, F. (2020). Italie: Vo'Euganeo, laboratoire de la quarantaine. *Libération*, 22 March.

De Sèze, C. (2020). Cinq hypothèses sur l'origine du Covid-19, de la plus sérieuse à la plus farfelue. *L'Express*, 19 April.

Dugit, F. (2020). Coronavirus: Cinq nouveaux cas en France, mais sans gravité. *Le Parisien*, 8 February.

Dupont, V. (2020). Coronavirus en Italie: Reportage exclusif au cœur de Bergame, la ville martyre qui ne compte plus ses morts. *RTBF*, 22 March.

Dutheil, G. (2020). Un premier cas de coronavirus détecté parmi les personnels de Roissy-Charles-de-Gaulle. *Le Monde*, 28 February.

Émilie, D., Humbert, M., Galanaud, P. (2020). Orage de cytokines: Quand le système immunitaire s'emballe. *Pour la Science*, 270.

ESA (2020). Plateforme Épidémiologie et Santé Animale [Online]. Available at: https://www.plateforme-esa.fr/#.

Faure, A. (2020). Coronavirus: Le match OL-Juventus a-t-il aggravé la situation? *Le Parisien*, 27 March.

Faure, Y. and Sciama, Y. (2021). Les élevages de visons en Chine à l'origine du Covid-19? Les preuves s'accumulent. *Reporterre*, 8 January.

Flaxman, S., Mishra, S., Gandy, A., Gandy, A., Unwin, H.J.T., Mellan, T.A., Coupland, H., Whittaker, C., Zhu, H., Berah, T., Eaton, J.W. (2020). Estimating the number of infections and the impact of non-pharmaceutical interventions on Covid-19 in 11 European countries. Imperial College, London.

Fontanet, A., Tondeur, L., Madec, Y., Grant, R., Besombes, C., Jolly, N., Pellerin, S.F., Ungeheuer, M.-N., Cailleau, I. (2020). Cluster of Covid-19 in northern France: A retrospective closed cohort study. *medRxiv*, 23 April.

Fraissard, G. (2004). Hôtel Métropole, chambre 911, l'histoire du SRAS. *Le Monde*, 28 February.

France info (2020a). Coronavirus: Qui sont les quatre victimes du Covid-19 en France? *France info*, 5 March.

France info (2020b). Covid-19: des zones de confinement dans l'Oise. *France info*, 1 March.

France info (2020c). Coronavirus: Sécurité, conditions de vie. Comment sont encadrés les Français placés en quarantaine à Carry-le-Rouet et à Aix-en-Provence? *France info*, 2 February.

France info (2020d). Coronavirus: Un rapatrié contaminé en Belgique. *France info*, 4 February.

France info (2020e). Covid-19: Une trentaine de Français rapatriés de Wuhan. *France info*, 21 February.

France info (2020f). Covid-19: Questions autour du décès d'une octogénaire de Crépy-en-Valois. *France info*, 3 March.

Fuhrmann, C. (2010). The effects of weather and climate on the seasonality of influenza: What we know and what we need to know. *Geography Compass*, 4, 718–730.

Gámbaro, F., Behillil, S., Baidaliuk, A., Donati, F., Albert, M., Alexandru, A., Vanpeene, M., Bizard, M., Brisebarre, A., Barbet, M. et al. (2020). Introductions and early spread of SARS-CoV-2 in France. *medRxiv*, 24 April.

Gardner, L., Zlojutro, A., Rey, D., Dong, E. (2020). Modeling the spread of 2019-nCoV. John Hopkins University [Online]. Available at: https://systems.jhu.edu/wp-content/uploads/2020/01/Gardner-JHU_nCoV-Modeling-Report_Jan-26.pdf.

Gerbaud, L., Guiguet-Auclair, C., Breysse, F., Odoul, J., Ouchchane, L., Peterschmitt, J., Dezfouli-Desfer, C., Breton, V. (2020). Hospital and population-based evidences for Covid-19 early circulation in the east of France? Preprints, 2020080204 [Online]. Available at: 10.20944/preprints202008.0204.v1.

Giordano, P. (2020). *Contagions*. Le Seuil, Paris.

Gleize, P. (2020). Coronavirus: La chaîne d'approvisionnement des médicaments remise en cause. *RFI*, 6 March.

Goffard, A. (2020). Que sait-on des mutations du SARS-CoV62 et de leurs effets? *The Conversation*, 13 September.

Goinère, G. (2020). Le quadragénaire atteint du coronavirus est sorti de l'hôpital. *Vitisphère*, 13 February.

Gourru, S. (2020a). Coronavirus: Le patient zéro de l'Oise est-il un militaire de la base de Creil? *Le Parisien*, 28 February.

Gourru, S. (2020b). Patient zéro dans l'Oise: Ni test biologique ni confinement pour les militaires de Creil revenus de Chine. *Le Parisien*, 2 March.

Guillot, M. and Khiat, M. (2020). Épidémie de Covid-19: Quel impact sur l'espérance de vie en France? *The Conversation*, 29 June.

Guimard, E. (2016). L'École des Mines de Nantes lance sa chaire sur les risques émergents. *Les Échos*, 5 April.

Haby, F. (2020). L'hôpital Schweitzer de Colmar évoque des cas de Covid dès novembre. *Dernières Nouvelles d'Alsace*, 7 May.

Hadjadj, J., Yatim, N., Barnabei, L., Corneau, A., Boussier, J., Smith, N., Péré, H., Charbit, B., Bondet, V., Chenevier-Gobeaux, C. et al. (2020). Impaired type I interferon activity and inflammatory responses in severe Covid-19 patients. *Science*, 369(6504), 718–724.

Han, J. and Kamber, M. (2006). *Data Mining: Concepts and Techniques*. Morgan Kaufmann Publishers, Burlington.

Haute Autorité de Santé (2020). Cahier des charges définissant les modalités d'évaluation des performances des tests sérologiques détectant les anticorps dirigés contre le SARS-CoV-2. Haute Autorité de Santé.

Herrero, O. (2020). Florence Parly admet finalement que les militaires de retour de Wuhan n'avaient pas été testés. *Capital*, 22 September.

Hiault, R. (2020). Coronavirus: La Banque mondiale alerte sur la remontée de l'extrême pauvreté. *Les Échos*, 7 October.

Hoffmann, M., Kleine-Weber, H., Schroeder, H., Krüger, N., Herrler, T., Erichsen, S., Schiergens, T.S., Herrler, G., Wu, N.H., Nitsche, A. et al. (2020). SARS-CoV-2 cell entry depends on ACE2 and TMPRSS2 and is blocked by a clinically proven protease inhibitor. *Cell*, 181(2), 271–280.

Hussain, M., Jabeen, N., Raza, F., Shabbir, S., Baig, A.A., Amanullah, A., Aziz, B. (2020). Structural variations in human ACE2 may influence its binding with SARS-CoV-2 spike protein. *Journal of Medical Virology* [Online]. Available at: https://doi.org/10.1002/jmv.25832.

Institut Pasteur (2020). L'Institut Pasteur séquence le génome complet du coronavirus SARS-CoV-2 [Online]. Available at: https://www.pasteur.fr/fr/espace-presse/documents-presse/institut-pasteur-sequence-genome-complet-du-coronavirus-sars-cov-2.

INVS (2011). La veille et l'alerte sanitaires en France. Institut de veille sanitaire, Saint-Maurice.

IRSN (2020). Le risque nucléaire et sa gestion [Online]. Available at: https://www.irsn.fr/FR/connaissances/Installations_nucleaires/La_surete_Nucleaire/risque-nucleaire/Pages/gestion-risque-nucleaire.aspx.

Islam, M.R., Hoque, M.N., Rahman, M.S., Rubayet Ul Alam, A.S.M., Akther, M., Akter Puspo, J., Akter, S., Sultana, M., Crandall, K.A., Anwar Hossain, M. (2020). Genome-wide analysis of SARS-CoV-2 virus strains circulating worldwide implicates heterogeneity. *Scientific Reports*, 10(14004) [Online]. Available at: https://doi.org/10.1038/s41598-020-70812-6.

Iwasaki, A. (2020). What reinfections means for Covid-19. *The Lancet Infectious Diseases* [Online]. Available at: https://doi.org/10.1016/S1473-3099(20)30783-0.

Johnson, R.M. and Vimetz, J.M. (2020). Dexamethasone in the management of Covid-19. *British Medical Journal*, 370 [Online]. Available at: https://doi.org/10.1136/bmj.m2648.

Jones, V.G., Mills, M., Suarez, D., Hogan, C.A., Yeh, D., Bradley Segal, J., Nguyen, E.L., Barsh, G.R., Maskatia, S., Mathew, R. (2020). Covid-19 and Kawasaki disease: Novel virus and novel case. *Hospital Pediatrics* [Online]. Available at: https://doi.org/10.1542/hpeds.2020-0123.

Jova, P. (2020). La Porte ouverte chrétienne, une Église souvent victime du lynchage médiatique. *La Vie*, 30 March.

Julien, E. (2020a). Coronavirus: Une centaine d'agents hospitaliers confinés à Compiègne et Creil. *Le Parisien*, 27 February.

Julien, E. (2020b). Coronavirus sur la base aérienne de Creil: Quand je demande des explications, on me répond secret-défense. *Le Parisien*, 30 March.

Korber, B., Fischer, W.M, Gnanakaran, S., Yoon, H., Theiler, J., Abfalterer, W., Hengartner, N., Giorgi, E.E., Bhattacharya, T. et al. (2020). Tracking changes in SARS-CoV-2 Spike: Evidence that D614G increases infectivity of the Covid-19 virus. *Cell*, 182(4), 812–827.

La Croix (2020a). Coronavirus: Ce que l'on sait sur le foyer de contamination dans l'Oise. *La Croix*, 28 February.

La Croix (2020b). Journée mondiale des femmes: L'Espagne défile contre le patriarcavirus. *La Croix*, 8 March.

Larousserie, D. (2020). Hubert Laude, virologue d'avant-garde. *Le Monde*, 6 April.

Lemke, C. (2020). Covid-19: Ce que l'on sait de la "molécule prometteuse" de l'Institut Pasteur de Lille. *Sciences et Avenir*, 1st October.

Le Parisien (2020a). Coronavirus: l'Italie décrète l'état d'urgence pour éviter une contagion. *Le Parisien*, 31 January.

Le Parisien (2020b). Coronavirus: Des fidèles contaminés partout en France après un rassemblement évangélique à Mulhouse. *Le Parisien*, 5 March.

Le Parisien (2020c). Coronavirus: Les organisateurs du rassemblement évangélique à Mulhouse se justifient. *Le Parisien*, 7 March.

Le Parisien (2020d). Coronavirus: 19 nouveaux cas en France, une étape est franchie. *Le Parisien*, 29 February.

L'Équipe (2020). Coronavirus: 35 % de cas positifs au Valence CF. *L'Équipe*, 16 March.

Liu, X., Goirgi, E.E., Honnayakanahalli Marichannegowda, M., Foley, B., Xiao, C., Kong, X.P., Chen, Y., Gnanakaran, S., Korber, B., Gao, F. (2020). Emergence of SARS-CoV-2 through recombination and strong purifying selection. *Science Advances*, 6(27), eabb9153.

Magal, M. (2020). Gestion de la Covid-19: Quelles leçons à tirer de Taiwan et de la Corée? *Public Sénat*, 9 September.

Mandl, J.N., Ahmed, R., Barreiro, L.B., Daszak, P. (2015). Reservoir host immune responses to emerging zoonotic viruses. *Cell*, 160(1–2), 20–35.

Mari, E. (2020). Coronavirus en France: D'autres patients pourraient sortir dans les prochains jours. *Le Parisien*, 12 February.

Martin, N. (2020). Coronavirus: La mutation continue. *France Culture*, 26 March.

McLean, S. and Feleke, B. (2020). One man linked to at least 9 coronavirus cases after traveling from Singapore to France to UK. *CNN*, 11 February.

Mei, T.T. and Taj, T.F. (2020). Coronavirus: Gas analysis conference at grand Hyatt Singapore linked to infections. *The Straits Times*, 7 February.

Mercier, A. (2020). La France en pénurie de masques: Aux origines des décisions d'État. *The Conversation*, 22 March.

Ministère des Armées (2018). L'escadron de transport aérien Estérel célèbre ses 50 ans. 9 October.

Ministère des Armées (2020a). Coronavirus Covid-19: Le Ministère des Armées démêle le vrai du faux. 16 March.

Ministère des Armées (2020b). L'armée de l'air au service des Français. 16 March.

Monteil, V., Kwon, H., Prado, P. et al. (2020). Inhibition of SARS-CoV-2 infections in engineered human tissues using clinical-grade soluble human ACE2Ast. *Cell*, 181.4.

Offord, C. (2017). Why Iceland is the world's greatest genetic laboratory. *The Scientist*, 1 June.

O'Malley, M.A. (2016). The ecological virus. *Studies in History and Philosophy of Science Part C: Studies in History and Philosophy of Biological and Biomedical Sciences*, 59, 71–79.

ONERC (2020). Observatoire national sur les effets du réchauffement climatique. Ministère de la Transition écologique et solidaire [Online]. Available at: https://www.ecologique-solidaire.gouv.fr/observatoire-national-sur-effets-du-rechauffement-climatique-onerc#e0.

Opoczinski, D. (2020). Covid-19: Des athlètes français contaminés à Wuhan en octobre? *Le Parisien*, 6 May.

Organisation Européenne et Méditerranéenne pour la Protection des Plantes (2020). Ecophytopic [Online]. Available at: https://ecophytopic.fr/pour-aller-plus-loin/organisation-europeenne-et-mediterraneenne-pour-la-protection-des-plantes-oepp.

Peffault de Latour, R., Bergeron, A., Lengline, E., Dupont, T., Marchal, A., Galicier, L., de Castro, N., Bondeelle, L., Darmon, M., Dupin, C. (2020). Complement C5 inhibition in patients with Covid-19 – A promising target? *Haematologica*, 105(12).

Piétri, J. (2020). À Mulhouse avec SOS Médecins: C'est peut-être le coronavirus, vous en avez les symptomes. *France inter*, 10 March.

Planetoscope (2020). Planetoscope. FACTOSOFT [Online]. Available at: https://www.planetoscope.com/mortalite.

Pouga, L. (2020). Infection par le SARS-CoV-2: Attention aux signes neurologiques! *La Revue du praticien*, 70(5), 532–535.

Préfecture du Haut-Rhin (2020). Coronavirus – Points de situation dans le Haut-Rhin. Préfecture du Haut-Rhin, February–March.

Riddell, S., Goldie, S., Hill, A., Eagles, D., Drew, T.W. (2020). The effect of temperature on persistence of SARS-CoV-2 on common surfaces. *Virology Journal*, 17(145).

Roy, S. (2020). Coronavirus: En France, un homme était déjà infecté fin décembre. *Le Figaro Santé*, 5 May.

R'Pro'Mobilité (2016). Domiciliation des salariés de la plateforme aéroportuaire Paris-Charles-de-Gaulle [Online]. Available at: https://www.rpromobilite.fr/nos-r%C3%A9alisations/etude-de-domiciliation/.

RTBF Info (2020). Le Belge contaminé par le coronavirus peut quitter l'hôpital Saint-Pierre. *RTBF Info*, 15 February.

Sache, I. and Barnouin, J. (eds) (2006). Méthodes et stratégies d'analyse épidémiologique des maladies émergentes chez le végétal, l'animal et l'homme. *Colloque Émergences*, Paris.

Sagar, M., Reifler, K., Rossi, M., Miller, N.S., Sinha, P., White, L.F., Mizgerd, J.P. (2020). Recent endemic coronavirus infection is associated with less severe Covid-19. *The Journal of Clinical Investigation*, 9 [Online]. Available at: https://www.jci.org/articles/view/143380.

Salje, H., Tran Kiem, C., Lefrancq, N., Courtejoie, N., Bosetti, P., Paireau, J., Andronico, A., Hozé, N., Richet, J., Dubost, C.-L. et al. (2020a). Estimating the burden of SARS-CoV-2 in France. *Science*, 369(6500), 208–211 [Online]. Available at: https://science.sciencemag.org/content/369/6500/208/tab-article-info.

Saltmarsh, A. (2020b). Coronavirus: How robots are helping fight the outbreak. *Direct Industry*, 11 February.

Sama, I.E., Ravera, A., Santema, B.T., van Goor, H., ter Maaten, J.M., Cleland, J.G.F., Rienstra, M., Friedrich, A.W., Samani, N.J., Ng, L.L. et al. (2020). Circulating plasma concentrations of angiotensin-converting enzyme 2 in men and women with heart failure and effects of renin–angiotensin–aldosterone inhibitors. *European Heart Journal*, 41(19), 1810–1817 [Online]. Available at: https://doi.org/10.1093/eurheartj/ehaa373.

Samama, P. (2020). Coronavirus: Air France suspend les vols vers Wuhan et réduit ceux vers Pékin et Shanghai. *BFM TV*, 29 January.

Sanche, S., Lin, Y.T., Xu C., Romero-Severson, E., Hengartner, N., Ke, R. (2020). High contagiousness and rapid spread of severe acute respiratory syndrome coronavirus 2. *Emerging Infectious Diseases*, 26(7).

Schulte-Schrepping, J., Reusch, N., Paclik, D., Baßler, K., Schlickeiser, S., Zhang, B., Krämer, B., Krammer, T., Brumhard, S., Bonaguro, L. et al. (2020). Severe Covid-19 is marked by a dysregulated myeloid cell compartment. *Cell* [Online]. Available at: https://doi.org/10.1016/j.cell.2020.08.001.

SGDN (2011). Plan national de Prévention et de lutte "Pandémie grippale", document d'aide à la préparation et à la décision, no. 850/SGDSN/PSE/PSN [Online]. Available at: https://solidarites-sante.gouv.fr/IMG/pdf/Plan_Pandemie_ Grippale_ 2011.pdf.

Société Française de Pharmacologie et de Thérapeutique (2020). ACE2, IEC/ARAII et infections à Covid-19 [Online]. Available at: https://www.elsevier.com/fr-fr/connect/medecine/ace2,-iecaraii-et-infections-a-covid-19.

Sud-Ouest (2020). Coronavirus: Deux enfants contaminés en Alsace, premiers cas en outre-mer. *Sud-Ouest*, 1 March.

Tang, X., Wu, C., Li, X., Song, Y., Yao, X., Wu, X., Duan, Y., Zhang, H., Wang, Y., Qian, Z. et al. (2020). On the origin and continuing evolution of SARS-CoV-2. *National Science Review* [Online]. Available at: https://doi.org/ 10.1093/nsr/nwaa036.

Tanguy, Y. (2020). Coronavirus: Un match de football responsable de l'épidémie en Italie? *RTL*, 24 March.

Tillett, R.L., Sevinsky, J.R., Hartley, P.D., Kerwin, H., Crawford, N., Gorzalski, A., Laverdure, C., Verma, S.C., Rossetto, C.C., Jackson, D. et al. (2020). Genomic evidence for reinfection with SARS-CoV-2: A case study. *The Lancet Infectious Diseases*, October 12.

Valentin, S., Arsevska, E., Falala, S., De Goër, J. (2020). PADI-web: A multilingual event-based surveillance system for monitoring animal infectious diseases. *Computers and Electronics in Agriculture*, 169.

Van der Made, C.I., Simons, A., Schuurs-Hoeijmakers, J., van den Heuvel, G., Mantere, T., Kersten, S., van Deuren, R.C., Steehouwer, M., van Reijmersdal, S.V., Jaeger, M. et al. (2020). Presence of genetic variants among young men with severe Covid-19. *Journal of American Medical Association*, 34(5), 663–673.

Vergnenère, A. (2020). Coronavirus: 35 nouveaux ressortissants français arrivés sur le site de l'Ensosp à Aix-en-Provence. *France 3 Provence-Alpes-Côte d'Azur*, 10 February.

Wang, C., Li, W., Drabek, D., Okba, N.M.A., van Haperen, R., Osterhaus, A.D.M.E., van Kuppeveld, F.J.M., B.L. Haagmans, Grosveld, F., Bosch, B.-J. (2020). A human monoclonal antibody blocking SARS-CoV-2 infection. *Nature Communications*, 11(2251).

Wu, Z. and McGoogan, J.M. (2020). Characteristics of and important lessons from the coronavirus disease 2019 (Covid-19) outbreak in China: Summary of a Report of 72 314 cases from the chinese centre for disease control and prevention. *Journal of the American Medical Association*, 323(13), 1239–1242.

Wu, Y., Jing, W., Liu, J., Ma, Q., Yuan, J., Wang, Y., Du, M., Liu, M. (2020). Effects of temperature and humidity on the daily new cases and new deaths of Covid-19 in 166 countries. *Science of The Total Environment*, 729.

Yahoo! Actualités (2020). Coronavirus: Au moins 1000 fidèles auraient été contaminés après le rassemblement évangélique de Mulhouse en février. *Yahoo! Actualités*, 28 March.

Yao, H., Lu, X., Chen, Q., Xu, K., Chen, Y., Cheng, L., Liu, F., Wu, Z., Wu, H., Jin, C. et al. (2020). Patient-derived mutations impact pathogenicity of SARS-CoV-2. *medRxiv*.

Zhou, G., Chen, S., Chen, Z. (2020). Advances in Covid-19: The virus, the pathogenesis, and evidence-based control and therapeutic strategies. *Frontiers of Medicine*, 1–9.

2

The Story of a Pandemic Foretold: Focus on the Covid-19 Vaccine

2.1. 2002, the first warning

In November 2002, cases of SARS appeared in Canton and later in Guangzhou, Beijing, Hanoi, Vietnam, Hong Kong and other cities in Southeast Asia. By May 2003, more than 8,000 people were reported to be ill and 700 to have died. The majority of those infected by the virus recover quickly, but some are subject to a worsening of the disease. Death (about 10% of patients) is generally linked to a cytokine storm leading to multivisceral failure (massive production of interleukin 6, TNF alpha and interleukin 12). The most pessimistic estimates predicted that 30% of the world's population would contract SARS. On April 16, 2003, the World Health Organization (WHO) announced that a new pathogen, a coronavirus never before seen in humans, was the causative agent of Severe Acute Respiratory Syndrome (SARS). At the end of April 2003, the genome of the new coronavirus (named SARS-CoV-1) was sequenced. Phylogenetically, SARS-CoV-1 is different from a known group of coronaviruses (HCoV) responsible for rhinopharyngitis – generally benign – that we have all encountered at some point. Some HCoVs, however, can occasionally cause acute respiratory distress and death while circulating in epidemic forms that are usually seasonal.

In view of the great flexibility of their genomes, their ability to cross species barriers, to adapt to humans and to establish persistent infections in

---

Chapter written by Jean-Pierre GIRARDEAU.

them, virologists and epidemiologists consider that coronaviruses should be monitored in order to rapidly identify the emergence of new viral strains that can cause severe infections. However, because the 2002–2003 SARS outbreak remained localized in southeastern China, this epidemic has been relatively forgotten.

One of the speakers at the *Émergences 2006* conference held in October 2006 in Paris, Arnaud Fontanet (Epidemiology of Emerging Diseases Unit, Pasteur Institute, Paris), anticipated in his presentation what would happen to us 14 years later (Fontanet 2006). In this text, everything was said, a passage from bats to civets in Chinese markets, then the adaptation to humans following the change of two amino acids of the S protein (spike protein) which allows the adhesion to the ACE2 receptor of the human respiratory epithelium. During the 2002–2003 episode, the human-to-human transmission of SARS-CoV-1 from infected animals (the civet?) must have been initially low, and therefore difficult to identify and trace, with a fraction of patients seemingly unable to transmit it (however, a few cases were at the origin of a large number of secondary cases, "super contaminators" or "super excretors"). Nevertheless, more than 8,000 SARS-CoV-1-related cases have been reported in 30 countries (of which nearly 20% were among caregivers), resulting in 774 deaths (about 10% mortality) (Peiris et al. 2004). The high contagiousness of SARS-CoV-1 was evident, as it was possible to link more than half of the infections a posteriori to a single patient who arrived in Hong Kong in February 2003 (Inserm 2015). The epidemic was brought under control by a global alert triggered by the WHO, which led to early detection of cases, isolation of patients at the onset of symptoms, management of contacts and protection of caregivers. It is likely that SARS-CoV-1 continues to spread – at a low level – between a host (probably a bat) and other intermediary animals in the direction of humans, but the absence of epidemiological surveillance makes it impossible to know how the disease is evolving. Apart from specialists, this first alert went unnoticed in the West. SARS was a problem of the distant and remote East.

2.2. 2012, a second warning

In 2012, 10 years after the SARS episode, another coronavirus respiratory syndrome (accompanied by vomiting, diarrhea and renal failure) developed in the Middle East and South Korea from Saudi Arabia (the virus responsible was named MERS-CoV). Death is, again, often linked to a cytokine storm (massive production of interleukin 6 and interleukins 1 and 8). The transmission of the virus continues today on a small scale, and a total of 2,519 cases and 867 deaths have been recorded in 27 countries (with a very high case-fatality rate of approximately 35%). In France, two cases were diagnosed in 2013 at the Lille University Hospital (Inserm 2015). The MERS-CoV virus, whose host also appears to be a bat, was probably transmitted to humans by an intermediate host, the dromedary, via urine, milk and saliva. Although the virus appears to have a low level of transmissibility, in May 2015, five super contaminators returning from the Middle East caused 154 infections and 35 deaths in South Korea (Korea Centers for Disease Control and Prevention 2015). Preventive measures implemented by the WHO, such as limiting contact with camels, masks for caregivers, hand washing and patient isolation, were effective in containing MERS-CoV infection. Curiously, the WHO did not recommend any restriction of travel (pilgrimage to Mecca) and trade, nor the implementation of screening procedures to prevent this infection. In the West, this second alert was hardly reported; MERS-CoV was for Saudi Arabia, with its deserts and its camels and so on.

Yet, from the laboratories, many virologists and epidemiologists warned "the zoonotic origin of SARS-CoV highlights the likelihood of re-emergence or evolution of new human coronaviruses" (Sui et al. 2014):

> The presence of a large reservoir of SARS-CoV-like viruses in horseshoe bats, together with the culture of eating exotic mammals in southern China, is a time bomb. The possibility of the re-emergence of SARS and other novel viruses from animals or laboratories and therefore the need for preparedness should not be ignored (Cheng et al. 2007).

Virologists and epidemiologists call for research efforts to be focused on the development of therapeutic or prophylactic measures ("since no vaccines for SARS-CoV-1 and MERS-CoV are currently available, preventive and therapeutic measures are urgently needed" (Kim 2019)). As early as October 2003, a future pandemic was announced at a symposium in Washington, D.C., entitled *Learning from SARS: Preparing for the Next Disease Outbreak* (Knobler *et al.* 2013).

These warnings have not really been heeded. Every day, we are told that we are caught off guard with this new virus, that we have everything to learn, that we are helpless and that we have to wait until we know how to solve the problem. Yet, the state of knowledge acquired since 2003 on SARS-CoV-1 and MERS-CoV (see the 4,000 publications available online as of 2007 (Cheng et al. 2007)) opened the door to the development of antivirals and vaccines proven in animal models (Hilgenfeld and Peiris 2013; Song 2019). However, in the end, like a tsunami that we watch coming towards us without running for cover on high ground, we waited for the wave, while we had time to escape it.

2.3. 2019, the pandemic

At the end of 2019, it was again "far from home" that a new episode in the evolution of coronaviruses took place. Thus, deep in China, a SARS-like cataclysm was set in motion, starting low-key, from – perhaps – a busy seafood market where live exotic animals were sold. Again, in the West we were initially looking at this episode from a distance, and on the other hand Chinese officials were reassuring. Everything seemed to be relatively under control and planes continued to pour thousands of Chinese tourists around the world, who were searching for knowledge of the world and financially attractive. However, in a period of a few weeks, the Wuhan district (11 million inhabitants) was submerged and thousands of cases of an atypical pneumopathy responsible for hundreds of deaths were announced. Here again, death was linked to a cytokine storm (massive production of interleukins 6, 2, 7 and 10, G-CSF, TNF alpha and interferon-induced proteins). Despite extreme containment measures, 2019 SARS spread first to China, then to South Korea and Iran and so on. In January 2020, the West woke up; this time the contagion spread rapidly. Luckily, however, the mortality rate was much lower than that seen throughout the MERS-CoV outbreak (2% vs. 30%).

The culprit of SARS-2019 (Covid-19) was quickly identified by Chinese virologists as a new SARS-CoV (the so-called SARS-CoV-2) very similar to SARS-CoV-1 from 2002. As in 2002, human-to-human transmission was initially weak, from infected animals, and therefore difficult to identify and trace. This time, the intermediate animal was initially identified as the Asian pangolin and the viral host a bat of the *Rhinolophus affinis* type (96% genetic similarity with SARS-CoV-2). Nevertheless, subsequent studies have not supported the pangolin hypothesis and the "intermediate animal" is still unknown. More importantly, virologists observed that the six amino acids of the receptor binding domain (RBD) of the virus' S protein involved in binding to human receptors are identical between *Rhinolophus affinis* CoV and SARS-CoV-2. If *Rhinolophus affinis* CoV was unsuitable for infection of human cells, it did have the key to enter them (Zhang et al. 2020). Nevertheless, subsequent events showed that the virus had refined its human-to-human transmission capabilities and spread rapidly worldwide via air travel, with the largest outbreaks concentrated in airport hubs. Within two months, a pandemic of exceptional magnitude developed via a well-known virus type and through apparently local epidemiological circumstances (Yi et al. 2020).

2.4. SARS-CoV-2: far from unknown

"Fortunately", the 2019 SARS-CoV-2 is very similar to the 2002 SARS-CoV-1 (89% genetic similarity) (Chen 2020b). Thanks to the work of virologists on these two viruses, progress on SARS-CoV-2 has been made fairly quickly. As early as January 10, 2020, Chinese researchers published the nucleotide sequence of the virus and identified the sequences of its various proteins. Very quickly, it was known that the S protein (which forms the characteristic spicules of coronaviruses) of SARS-CoV-2 uses the same receptor on human cells as SARS-CoV-1 (in this case, ACE2, angiotensin-converting enzyme 2). The experience of clinicians – and the extensive scientific work done over the past 18 years on SARS-CoV-1 – has helped with the management of Covid-19 patients and has saved time in tailoring treatments (choice of antivirals and immune regulators). Despite this, Covid-19 takes its toll.

Studies on the structures and functions of SARS-CoV-1 proteins have been used in the design of new antivirals and a vaccine against SARS-CoV-2. Typically, it takes many years to develop safe and effective therapies and vaccines. In the short term, however, vaccine candidates can be tested in humans within a few months.

The ability of SARS coronaviruses to cross the species barrier is a major factor in the amplification of viral pathogens from host species (probably bats) to intermediate species and then to humans. Genetic mutations and rearrangements probably facilitated this interspecies transmission, allowing the virus to be recognized by receptors on the surface of cells of different hosts. Apparently, small changes (two amino acid residues) in the receptor site of the SARS-CoV-1 spike (S) protein allowed adaptation from civet to humans, and with SARS-CoV-2, new mutations allowed adaptation to humans and then inter-human transmission.

The S protein is a viral fusion protein that self-associates into trimers on the surface of the virus and recognizes the angiotensin-2-converting enzyme as a fusion receptor. The association with the cellular receptor allows the insertion of a fusion peptide present on the S protein and leads to entry of the virus into the cell via fusion between the cell membrane and the viral envelope. Interestingly, sequence analysis indicates that SARS-CoV-2 has an insertion of a furin cleavage site in its spike protein. Absent in SARS-CoV-1 and MERS-CoV, the insertion of a furin cleavage site may be a key factor in the replication and virulence of SARS-CoV-2. Interactions with different signaling pathways in the host cell (induction of apoptosis, production of inflammatory cytokines) are also associated with the S-ACE2 protein present on the cells of the pulmonary epithelium as well as on other tissues (nose, tongue, oesophagus, intestine, kidney), which explains why SARS-CoV-2 targets organs other than the lungs. Moreover, the S proteins of SARS-CoV-1 and SARS-CoV-2 are very similar (80% homology in protein sequence), with high homology of the fusion site with ACE2 (Du et al. 2009; Sui et al. 2014; Kim et al. 2019; Song 2019).

2.5. Vaccine design possible as early as 2010

Despite the 2002–2003 SARS episode, there is still no vaccine against SARS-CoV-1. However, since then, a lot of work has been done on the immunogenicity of SARS-CoV proteins (SARS-CoV-1 and MERS) and on vaccine design (resulting in hundreds of publications). Thus, many candidate vaccines targeting SARS-CoV-1 proteins have been designed and studied: subunit vaccines using recombinant proteins (mostly directed against the S protein, to block binding with the ACE2 receptor); live attenuated virus vaccines; vaccines using recombinant viral vectors (measles vaccine virus, adenovirus, attenuated influenza), genetically modified to produce SARS-CoV-1 proteins; and DNA (deoxyribonucleic acid) or RNA (ribonucleic acid) vaccines (Chen 2020b). Among all the vaccine candidates, a subunit anti-SARS-CoV-1 protein vaccine appeared promising. Its design is described below.

Research on SARS-CoV-1 had shown that the S protein was the main antibody-inducing protein and, for this reason, was considered a major target for vaccine design (Du et al. 2009; Sui et al. 2014; Kim et al. 2019; Song 2019). As early as 2004, work on SARS-CoV-1 showed that animals immunized with whole viral vectors (baculovirus, adenovirus, attenuated influenza virus, measles vaccine virus), genetically engineered to express the S protein, developed high titers of anti-S antibodies, with potent neutralizing activities against different virus variants (Bukreyev et al. 2004). These vaccines had the advantage of eliciting a good immune response, but sometimes raised significant safety concerns. Some laboratory animals vaccinated with viral vectors expressing the S protein showed after challenge with a strain of SARS-CoV-1 an exacerbation of the disease (immunopotentiation) and immunopathological complications (Chen 2020b). Obviously, the fact that there are safety concerns for a vaccine complicates its development. Fortunately, an alternative approach of using only the receptor binding domain (RBD) of the S protein provided neutralizing antibodies and protective cellular immunity in vaccinated animals, while significantly reducing or eliminating disease immuno-potentiation and immuno-pathology issues (Jiang et al. 2012; Chen 2020b). Expressed and produced in yeast, the researchers identified a recombinant RBD of 219 AA residues (RBD219-N1) inducing strong humoral and cellular immunity, capable of neutralizing the virus in immune mice when adjuvanted with aluminum hydroxide (low immunopathological risk and development of memory lymphocytes). After optimizing the production and purification of RBD219-N1, the authors showed that the peptide retained the native conformation of RBD. The process had been transferred in 2016 to a pilot manufacturing plant as part of good drug substance manufacturing practices and the RBD219-N1 vaccine was to be used in a phase 1 clinical trial (Cheng et al. 2017). With the control of SARS episodes likely moving this goal to a lower priority, the development of this vaccine did not proceed and there was no phase 1 clinical trial.

The irony is that the same authors (Chen et al. 2020a) are now, four years later, proposing to reconsider the use of RBD219-N1 from SARS-CoV-1 as a heterologous vaccine against SARS-CoV-2. Indeed:

– serum from convalescent SARS-CoV-1 patients neutralizes SARS-CoV-2;

– SARS-CoV-1/SARS-CoV-2 protein sequence comparisons show high similarity (82%) of RBDs, and both RBDs bind to the same angiotensin-converting enzyme (ACE) 2 receptor;

– neutralizing monoclonal antibodies (mabs) to the RBD of SARS-CoV-1 target highly conserved regions (94% similarity) in the RBDs of SARS-CoV-1 and SARS-CoV-2.

Based on these observations, a recombinant subunit vaccine designed with the RBD219-N1 peptide offered the potential to develop a SARS-CoV-2 vaccine. In addition, a substantial improvement could be rapidly achieved by replacing RBD219 SARS-CoV-1 with RBD219 SARS-CoV-2. The safety and efficacy of the vaccine candidate remain to be confirmed with human clinical trials. In addition, Covid-19 preferentially affects the elderly and those with co-morbidities such as diabetes and hypertension. It will also be important to ensure that in this population the vaccine will be effective and, more importantly, well tolerated (Chen et al. 2020b). In November 2020, the RBD219-N1C1 recombinant subunit vaccine was transferred to Biological E. Limited, an India-based vaccine and pharmaceutical company, and a phase I/II clinical trial was initiated in November 2020 in India. Four formulations are currently (January 2021) being evaluated to select the final vaccine candidate to be tested in subsequent phase III trials. Potential advantages of this vaccine candidate include scalability and thermostability, which could make it suitable for deployment at scale in low-resource settings. The induction of an improved immunity and neutralizing response should place RBD vaccines at a competitive position to provide a response against the SARS-CoV-2 pandemic. If the development of the RBD219-N1 vaccine had not been prematurely halted in 2016, it is likely that a SARS-CoV-2 RBD vaccine could have been available by 2020.

In the course of 2020, it was proposed to use antibodies from convalescent SARS-CoV-2 patients as immunotherapies for Covid-19 patients. The procedure has been proven successful on some occasions, but it involves risks of contamination with unknown infectious agents (e.g. prions), as well as problems with collection and mass purification of antibodies. A safe alternative is to use monoclonal antibodies, the industrial production of which is well controlled. In oncology, specific humanized mouse monoclonal antibodies (mabs) are routinely infused into patients to block membrane receptors (they are part of many commonly used targeted therapies). It has been known since the early 2000s that mouse mabs specific for the SARS-CoV-1 RBD fusion site had potent neutralizing activity and were able to block viral binding to receptors, confirming that the fusion site contained the major neutralizing epitopes and that receptor blockade was the primary mechanism of SARS-CoV-1 neutralization (Coughlin 2012). Specific mabs of the S protein fusion site could have been prepared for administration to patients with severe SARS. This approach, however, may have risks (such as immuno-potentiation of the disease) and has been explored and proven in animal models. In the course of 2020, this technology was redesigned for SARS-CoV-2 immunotherapy, and in November 2020, Donald Trump was able to benefit from monoclonal antibody treatment developed by the US firm Regeneron. Recently (August 2021), the FDA authorized a combination treatment of two monoclonal antibodies (casirivimab and imdevimab) to reduce Covid-19-related hospitalization and deaths in high-risk patients. When given to an exposed person, like someone living with an infected person, monoclonal antibodies reduced their risk of developing an infection with symptoms by 80%.

2.6. Lack of a vaccine: a collective responsibility

Collectively, national and international health policy and research bodies ignored previous warnings. They either did not identify the pandemic threats posed by SARS-CoV or assumed that they could control the spread of the virus through standard epidemic management measures.

Following the MERS-2012 outbreak, the WHO Director-General convened an emergency committee to assess whether this event constituted a public health emergency of international concern and to make recommendations on public health measures to be implemented. Among other things, it was to encourage WHO Member States to:

– strengthen their surveillance of severe acute respiratory infections (SARI);

– carefully examine any unusual presentation of SARS or pneumonia cases and report all confirmed and probable cases to WHO, with information on sources of exposure, tests performed and clinical course, to guide international preparedness and response and ensure its effectiveness.

In 2002 in China, in 2012 in the Middle East and in 2015 in South Korea, these measures were sufficient to control the spread of the virus. So, we could continue as before.

The mistake (fault?) was not supporting the design and production of vaccines, despite the warnings of scientists. Vaccination policy is the responsibility of public authorities, who commission independent scientific experts to define the relevant vaccinations. The pharmaceutical industry, on the other hand, does not start producing a vaccine without the encouragement and support of national or international public authorities. Indeed, for the pharmaceutical industry, the sale of drugs and parapharmaceuticals is far more profitable than the sale of vaccines. Since their production is often more complex and expensive than that of other pharmaceutical products, there are fewer and fewer vaccine manufacturers in the world.

For years, the accumulated knowledge of SARS-CoV-1 and MERS-CoV has enabled the design of vaccine candidates and the evaluation of their efficacy and safety (Cheng et al. 2007). In the Middle East, vaccination of camels, the intermediate hosts of MERS-CoV, was considered. A veterinary vaccine would have probably blocked transmission to humans by reducing camel carriage of the virus and would have provided a large-scale test of the efficacy and safety of a SARS-CoV vaccine. For example, it would have tested the level of risk of disease immunopotentiation and immunopathology associated with the vaccine in camels. Unfortunately, this project did not proceed.

In 2009, most industrialized countries feared the emergence of an influenza pandemic due to the H5N1 avian virus. Vaccines were developed on this principle, and as soon as the pandemic virus emerged, the "prototype" vaccine strain was replaced by the pandemic virus strain, thus shortening the production and marketing authorization times. Obviously, we are far from mastering the development and production technology for SARS-CoV as we have for influenza vaccines. However, so-called "prototype" vaccines designed against SARS-CoV-1 in 2002 could have been tested in animal models to test their efficacy and safety (some candidate vaccines have indeed led to an exacerbation of the disease). As discussed in 2016 with some vaccine candidates, phase 1 clinical studies could have been conducted with the most promising candidates. On the prototype vaccine principle, as soon as a new SARS-CoV emerged, the antigens or antigen parts of the prototype vaccine were replaced with the antigens or antigen parts of the emerging virus (with the vaccine proposed in 2016 by W. H. Chen, for example, RBD219 of SARS-CoV-1 was replaced with RBD219 of SARS-CoV-2). Since this strategy has not been adopted, everything remains to be done. Phase 1, 2 and 3 clinical trials will not be dispensed with. Then, we will have to move to production of the successful vaccine, which will take months or years. By that time, it is likely – and desirable – that the Covid-19 episode will be over. In that situation, will governments support the massive and costly production of a vaccine to control a past pandemic? However, we should exercise caution, if a vaccine strategy is not available in the next coronavirus pandemic, we will surely fall back into the same chaos we are experiencing at the time of writing (Chen 2020b).

2.7. SARS-CoV vaccinology: a pathway for rapid development of Covid-19 vaccines

Covid-19 is still rampant in many countries as we enter the year 2021. In the absence of decisive progress in antiviral therapies and faced with the possibility of a second wave in Europe, laboratories are working hard to develop a vaccine against SARS-CoV-2. The abundance of vaccine candidates (26 in clinical trials and 139 in pre-clinical evaluation) and the speed of their development may come as a surprise, given that the period between development and commercialization of a vaccine is usually long (15–20 years). However, as noted above, the development of these "new" vaccine candidates is based on the 15 years of SARS-CoV research. For example, a search of the main medical literature database (PubMed) – over a 14-year period prior to the Covid-19 pandemic – reveals 1,678 references. There is therefore no final reason to be surprised. Indeed, a decade ago, some SARS-CoV-1 and MERS-CoV vaccine candidates were already close to clinical trials. Following the "disappearance" of SARS-CoV-1 (2003 in China) and the lack of funding for research on this coronavirus, vaccine research against SARS-CoV-1 has unfortunately been exhausted (despite the warnings of researchers). In contrast, research into MERS-CoV (which was present in the Middle East in 2012) was still active in 2019, and it is in this area that the most recent advances have been made. Thus, the current Covid-19 vaccines on offer are not creations ex nihilo. The design of these vaccines is based on years of research in anti-SARS-CoV vaccinology that have resulted in:

– the identification of the S protein as the major inducer of neutralizing antibodies capable of blocking binding to the ACE2 receptor and mediating a specific T cell response;

– the study in detail of the vaccine response and demonstration of the crucial role of a T cell response in protection and long term memory;

– identification, analysis and problem solving with regard to vaccine immunopathology in animals;

– the clear identification of the type of immune response and vaccine procedures to avoid these problems (in response to a Th1 cell-mediated response that directs the body's reaction to produce interferon, a high level of high-affinity antibodies and a cytotoxic T8 cell response).

This Th1-type orientation of the vaccine response is one of the key Food and Drug Administration (FDA) recommendations on the development of a vaccine against Covid-19[1].

More than 20 years ago, the idea was already emerging to design a new class of vaccine based on DNA nucleic acids or messenger RNA (mRNA) encoding viral antigens (HIV, Zika, influenza). In 2015, a pre-clinical trial of a DNA vaccine (GLS-5300 encoding S protein) already showed a protective effect in monkeys after infection with MERS-CoV. In early 2019, a phase I trial launched by the Walter Reed Army Institute of Research Clinical Trials Center showed that GLS-5300 resulted in the production of neutralizing antibodies and a specific T cell response (Modjarrad et al. 2019).

From 2015 onwards, significant innovations in mRNA vaccine design, in particular the use of modified mRNAs encapsulated in lipid nanoparticles, have led to the emergence of a new generation of safe and effective vaccines (Sahin et al. 2014; Reichmuth et al. 2016; Pardin et al. 2017). For example, prototype vaccines developed from mRNAs encoding the MERS-CoV S protein served as a model for the development of the Pfizer–BioNTech and Moderna SARS-CoV-2 mRNA vaccines (Corbett et al. 2020).

---

1 For more information, please visit: https://www.fda.gov/regulatory-information/search-fda-guidance-documents/development-and-licensure-vaccines-prevent-covid-19.

2.8. Finalized and planned vaccines

Today, in the face of the health emergency, governments and laboratories are rushing to slow down the rate of infection. As a result, 172 countries have held discussions to participate in Covax, a global initiative to work with vaccine manufacturers to ensure that all countries have equitable access to safe and effective vaccines, once licensed and approved. Today, USD 6 billion is committed to vaccine research and development. A collaboration between the Serum Institute of India (SII), the Gavi Alliance and the Bill and Melinda Gates Foundation, through the Covax scheme, is expected to procure up to 100 million doses of the candidate vaccines, if successful, for low-income countries at USD 3 per dose. The goal of Covax is to provide 2 billion doses of safe and effective vaccines licensed by regulatory agencies and/or prequalified by WHO by the end of 2021. Vaccine candidates supported for development by the Covax mechanism include Inovio, USA (phase 1/2); Moderna, USA (phase 3); CureVac, Germany (phase 1); Institut Pasteur-Merck-Themis, France–USA–Austria (inconclusive preclinical trials); AstraZeneca–University of Oxford, UK (phase 3); University of Hong Kong, China (preclinical trials); Novavax, USA (phase 1/2); Clover Biopharmaceuticals, China (phase 1) and University of Queensland–CSL, Australia (phase 1). In addition to the vaccine candidates supported through Covax, there are so many vaccines under investigation, but their sponsors are not forthcoming about the strategies being used. Let us hope that in the rush, the lessons learned from the many research studies on SARS and MERS are not forgotten. Incomplete success of the vaccine strategy, for example, due to the diversity of SARS-CoV-2 strains, would be problematic and would give rise to the possibility that the vaccine could be used in a different way and would go some way to vindicating the anti-vaccine movements that speculate about its ineffectiveness, dangerousness and mandatory nature.

In October 2020, the *New England Journal of Medicine* reported in a first publication the main data obtained in a phase I/II study with the Pfizer/BioNTech mRNA vaccine tested on 195 participants in two age groups (18–55 and 65–85). Humoral and cellular responses were a Th1 cell-mediated response with high interferon-γ production and a CD8 T cell response. In this trial, no serious adverse events were observed. As expected, the vaccine response in the 65–85 age group was slightly lower than that in the 18–55 age group. However, as the level of neutralizing antibodies obtained with the 65–85 age group remained clearly higher than that observed in convalescents after Covid-19, a satisfactory protective effect was expected for this age group (Wal 2020; Sahin et al. 2020). Since then, we have learned that a phase III trial conducted on 43,000 volunteers confirmed the efficacy of the Pfizer–BioNTech vaccine (more than 94% protection) in all age groups (Pop 2020).

On December 15, 2020, Moderna released a briefing paper on the phase II/III trial of the mRNA-1273 vaccine (30,418 participants, with a follow-up time of 50 days after the first injection) (Bad 2020). The protection rate, estimated at 80% at one month after the first injection, increased to 94% at 14 days after the second injection. The results presented suggest efficacy against severe forms of Covid-19, but the immunogenicity and protection data for people with comorbidities are less convincing than for the Pfizer–BioNTech vaccine. Unlike the Pfizer–BioNTech vaccine, which requires storage at –70°C, the Moderna vaccine formulation, which allows storage at only –20°C, should provide more flexibility in meeting the organizational needs of vaccination centers. The short-term toxicity profile of mRNA vaccines is reassuring, with essentially the same reactions as those usually observed after vaccination: fatigue, headaches, aches and pains, chills, joint pain and fever, all of which subside rapidly. However, questions remain about the duration of immunity and transmission of the virus by vaccinated individuals. While the data presented seem to justify an emergency release of this vaccine, a post-vaccination surveillance system is planned to compensate for the short follow-up time of mRNA vaccines.

Astra Zeneca and the University of Oxford are proposing a vaccine based on a conventional technology, the injection of a non-replicating chimpanzee adenovirus genetically modified to produce the S protein of SARS-CoV-2. Despite relatively small and inaccurate clinical trials (70–90% protection), the UK Medicines Agency gave the green light – on December 30, 2020 – to this vaccine, making the United Kingdom the first country in the world to authorize it. The availability of AstraZeneca's vaccine appears crucial to the success of the vaccination campaign – in Europe as well as in the United States – since the manufacturing technique of this vaccine makes it much easier to produce, to store (2–8°C is sufficient), to distribute and to pay for (in Europe, EUR 1.78 per unit, compared with EUR 12 for the Pfizer–BioNTech vaccine and EUR 14.68 for the Moderna vaccine). This price is all the lower because AstraZeneca has pledged not to make any profit on its vaccine while the pandemic is ongoing. Thus, Europeans are counting on the arrival of AstraZeneca's vaccine to boost their vaccination campaigns. As a result, by the end of January 2021, 20 million people worldwide had been vaccinated against Covid-19, with efforts through hospitals, clinics, clinics, vaccination centers, special locations in urban areas and doctors' offices, pharmacists, nurses and other health professionals increasing daily.

Currently, a dozen candidate vaccines (using similar vaccine technologies) are in large phase III clinical trials (over 10,000 participants) involving more than 200,000 participants worldwide. The efficacy results of these vaccines are expected soon. The Food and Drug Administration in the United States and the European Medicines Agency in Europe remain vigilant, and marketing authorization will only be granted once it is certain that there will be no serious side effects following vaccination. The FDA's recommendations on the development of a vaccine against Covid-19 can be viewed online[2].

2.9. Conclusion: viral aggressor and human disruptor

The Covid-19 pandemic must serve as a major warning calling on the international community to support epidemiological research as a priority through:

– the identification of potential hosts, intermediate hosts and mechanisms of transmission of coronaviruses to humans;

– the development of global alert tools for all emerging diseases, such as emergences2 (see Chapter 1).

It will also be necessary, of course, to develop basic research in virology and immunology and also to promote prophylactic and therapeutic measures as a matter of urgency, with sufficient financial resources. If this proves possible, we should probably move towards the design of "pan-coronavirus" vaccines, followed – without delay – by human clinical trials. This pandemic may have had the merit of making us aware that the constant human flows across the planet make us particularly vulnerable to the risks of transmission of emerging infectious agents and that, in the absence of a vaccine, the control of zoonotic agents is still as uncontrollable as it has been in the past centuries.

2 See https://www.fda.gov/regulatory-information/search-fda-guidance-documents/development-and-licensure-vaccines-prevent-covid-19.

Many bio-tech companies have played a significant role in the fight against the Covid-19 pandemic, mainly in vaccines research and development. Significant financial efforts have helped to unlock the potential of RNA use in medicine, especially in mRNA vaccine development. In fact, mRNA vaccines are building on decades of scientific research. Recent technological advances, in particular modification of synthetic mRNA and lipid nanoparticles-based drug delivery systems, made these vaccines possible. Research on the SARS-CoV-2 S' protein made these mRNA vaccines effective. Beyond the mRNA Covid-19 vaccines, multiple mRNA vaccine platforms against infectious diseases and several types of cancer have demonstrated encouraging results in animal models and humans. Although the Covid-19 pandemic has harmed health, societies and economies worldwide, we can say that this crisis opened a new era in vaccine technology with promising potential for use in new medicines and therapies.

When we look at the ecology of the health of living organisms, we notice that human interventions are almost always at the origin of disturbances in ecosystems. So-called emerging or invasive species (plants, insects, parasites bacteria, viruses) were not in their original ecosystem, which controlled their development. The globalization of trade in goods and people has allowed the introduction into new ecosystems of intruders imported "accidentally" from their original ecosystem. The Covid-19 pandemic is not a health crisis, as people like to say, but an environmental crisis. The SARS episodes are a dramatic consequence of the inconsistency of *sapiens*. If humans had not disturbed the habitat of coronavirus-carrying bats, and if airplanes had not so easily transported millions of humans across the planet without due care, the coronavirus that caused Covid-19 might have quietly continued its life in bats, and we humans could still hug our children and loved ones without risking a stay in intensive care.

2.10. References

Al-Tawfiq, J.A., Zumla, A., Memish, Z.A. (2014). Travel implications of emerging coronaviruses: SARS and MERS-CoV. *Travel Medicine and Infectious Disease*, 12, 422–428.

Baden, L.R., El Sahly, H.M., Essink, B. et al. (2020). Efficacy and safety of the mRNA-1273 SARS-CoV-2 vaccine. *New England Journal of Medicine*, December 30.

Bukreyev, A., Lamirande, E.W., Buchholz, U.J. et al. (2004). Mucosal immunisation of African green monkeys (*Cercopithecus aethiops*) with an attenuated parainfluenza virus expressing the SARS coronavirus spike protein for the prevention of SARS. *Lancet*, 363, 2122–2127.

Chean, Y.Y., Ong, H.K., Yeap, S.K., Ho, K.L. (2019). Recent advances in the vaccine development against Middle East respiratory syndrome-coronavirus. *Frontiers in Microbiology*, 10, 1781.

Chen, W.H., Chag, S.M., Poongavanam, M.V. et al. (2017). Optimization of the production process and characterization of the yeast-expressed SARS-CoV recombinant receptor-binding domain (RBD219-N1), a SARS vaccine candidate. *Journal of Pharmaceutical Sciences*, 106, 1961–1970.

Chen, W.H., Hotez, P.J., Bottazzi, M.E. (2020a). Potential for developing the SARS-CoV receptor binding domain recombinant protein (RBD) as a heterologous human vaccine for SARS-CoV-2. *Human Vaccine Immunotherapy*, 16, 1–4.

Chen, W.H., Strych, U., Hotez, P.J., Bottazzi, M.E. (2020b). The SARS-CoV-2 vaccine pipeline: An overview. *Current Tropical Medicine Report*, March 3.

Cheng, V.C.C., S.K.P., Lau, P.C.Y., Woo, K.Y., Yuen (2007). Severe acute respiratory syndrome coronavirus as an agent of emerging and reemerging infection. *Clinical Microbiology Reviews*, 20, 660–694.

Corbett, K.S., Edwards, D.K., Leist, S.R. et al. (2020). SARS-CoV-2 mRNA vaccine design enabled by prototype pathogen preparedness. *Nature*, 586, 567–571.

Coughlin, M.M. and Prabhakar, B.S. (2012). Neutralizing human monoclonal antibodies to severe acute respiratory syndrome coronavirus: Target, mechanism of action, and therapeutic potential. *Reviews in Medical Virology*, 2, 2–17.

De Wit, E., van Doremalen, N., Falzarano, D., Munster, V.J. (2016). SARS and MERS: Recent insights into emerging coronaviruses. *Nature Reviews Microbiology*, 14, 523–534.

Du, L., He, Y., Zhou, Y., Liu, S. et al. (2009). The spike protein of SARS-CoV – A target for vaccine and therapeutic development. *Nature Reviews Microbiology*, 7, 226–236.

Fontanet, A. (2006). Les maladies émergentes chez l'homme: Les exemples du SRAS et de la grippe aviaire. *Colloque Émergences*, Paris, 26–27.

Hilgenfeld, R. and Peiris, M. (2013). From SARS to MERS: 10 years of research on highly pathogenic human coronaviruses. *Antiviral Research*, 100, 286–295.

Inserm (2015). Comprendre les coronavirus. L'épidémie de Syndrome respiratoire aigu sévère (SRAS-CoV) [Online]. Available at: https://www.inserm.fr/information-en-sante/dossiers-information/coronavirus-sars-cov-et-mers-cov.

Jiang, S., Bottazzim, M.E., Du, L. et al. (2012). Roadmap to developing a recombinant coronavirus S protein receptor-binding domain vaccine for severe acute respiratory syndrome. *Expert Review of Vaccines*, 11, 1405–1413.

Kim, M.H., Kim, H.J., Chang, J. (2019). Superior immune responses induced by intranasal immunization with recombinant adenovirus-based vaccine expressing full-length spike protein of Middle East respiratory syndrome coronavirus. *PLoS One*, 14, e0220196.

Knobler, S., Mahmoud, A., Lemon, S., Mack, A., Sivitz, L., Oberholtzer, K. (eds) (2003). *Learning from SARS: Preparing for the Next Disease Outbreak*. Smithsonian S. Dillon Ripley Center, Washington, D.C., 30 September–1 October.

Korea Centers for Disease Control and Prevention (2015). Middle East respiratory syndrome coronavirus outbreak in the Republic of Korea. *Osong Public Health and Research Perspectives*, 6, 269–278.

Liu, W.J., Zhao, M., Liu, K. et al. (2017). T-cell immunity of SARS-CoV: Implications for vaccine development against MERS-CoV. *Antiviral Research*, 137, 82–92.

Modjarrad, K., Roberts, C.C., Mills, K.T. et al. (2019). Safety and immunogenicity of an anti-Middle East respiratory syndrome coronavirus DNA vaccine: A phase 1, open-label, single-arm, dose-escalation trial. *The Lancet Infectious Diseases*, 19, 1013–1022.

Pardi, N., Hogan, M.J., Porter, F.W. et al. (2017). mRNA vaccines – A new era in vaccinology. *Nature Reviews Drug Discovery*, 4, 261–279.

Peiris, J.S.M., Guan, Y., Yuen, K.Y. (2004). Sever acute respiratory syndrome. *Nature Medecine*, 10, S88–S97.

Polack, F.P., Thomas, S.J., Kitchin, N. et al. (2020). Safety and efficacy of the BNT162b2 mRNA Covid-19 vaccine. *New England Journal of Medicine*, 27, 2603–2615.

Reichmuth, A.M., Oberli, M.A., Jaklenec, A. et al. (2016). mRNA vaccine delivery using lipid nanoparticles. *Therapeutic Delivery*, 7, 319–334.

Robin, C. (2020). Covid-19: Où en sont les vaccins? *Capital* [Online]. Available at: https://www.capital.fr/economie-politique/covid-19-ou-en-sont-les-vaccins-1382540.

Roper, R.L. and Rehm, K.E. (2009). SARS vaccines: Where are we? *Travel Medicine and Infectious Disease*, 12, 422–428.

Sahin, U., Karikó, K., Türeci, Ö. (2014). mRNA-based therapeutics – Developing a new class of drugs. *Nature Reviews Drug Discovery*, 10, 759–780.

Song, Z. (2019). From SARS to MERS, thrusting coronaviruses into the spotlight. *Viruses*, 14, 11–17.

Sui, J., Deming, M., Rockx, B. et al. (2014). Effects of human anti-spike protein receptor binding domain antibodies on severe acute respiratory syndrome coronavirus neutralization escape and fitness. *Journal of Virology*, 88, 13769–13780.

Walsh, E.E., Frenck Jr., R.W., Falsey, A.R. et al. (2020). Safety and immunogenicity of two RNA-based Covid-19 vaccine candidates. *NEJM*, 25, 2439–2450.

Yi, Y., Lagniton, P., Ye, S. et al. (2020). Covid-19: What has been learned and to be learned about the novel coronavirus disease. *International Journal of Biological Science*, 16, 1753–1766.

Zhang, T., Wu, Q., Zhang, Z. (2020). Probable pangolin origin of SARS-CoV-2 associated with the Covid-19 outbreak. *Current Biology*, 30, 1346–1351.

3

Remote Working after Lockdown

3.1. Elements in the development of remote working

In order to quickly adapt to the Covid-19 crisis, many companies set up remote working solutions (professional activity carried out entirely or partly remotely from the place where the result of the work is expected), as an emergency for some and with a procedure studied on the occasion of the 2009 A-H1N1 flu epidemic for others.

Curiously, remote working was introduced quietly, as a non-event. It could be said that it was taken for granted. Yet, in the 25 years since they first appeared in France, remote communication technologies have made meteoric progress. Broadband coverage in France is very significant. Thus, in the 4th quarter of 2019, 99.5% of French homes had access to the Internet, with 66.6% eligible for very high speed (>30 Mb/s or megabits per second) and 49.8% eligible for the fiber-optic network. Several operators have also launched 4G boxes that amplify the 4G signal (the fourth generation of cell phone standards) in homes with poor broadband coverage.

It should be remembered that in 1995, according to UFB-Locabail, 7% of SMEs–SMIs (small- and medium-sized enterprises–small- and medium-sized industries) had access to the Internet in France and, according to the *Association des professionnels de l'information et de la documentation* (ADBS), 15% of information professionals used it, while at the time there were only 370,000 computers in homes.

Chapter written by Emmanuel MIGNOT.

Moreover, the average price of a personal computer went from FRF 35,000 (EUR 5,335) in 1990 to FRF 17,400 (EUR 2,652) in 1994, and is now around EUR 460. Moreover, the performances are no longer at all the same, neither for the networks nor for the hardware. In 1995, the modems available allowed a speed of 2,400 BPS (number of bits transmitted in one second), which meant that the display of a simple page of text was not instantaneous; and for an image, you had to be patient.

We can be surprised that so many people made so much effort to join the computer adventure. Especially since at the time, there was no forum for mutual help, and the concept of a hotline did not exist. What was proposed by the manufacturers was both indigent and overpriced, and you had to take out an annual subscription. As for the cost of the computer connection, it was also very high, just like the telephone.

In 1986, at the first *Cité de la réussite* held at the Sorbonne (Paris), Robert Maxwell explained: “When I’m sitting at a café, this table becomes my office.” This was a real revelation! Thirty-four years later, the idea has made its way, it crossed the winter of 1999 and its strikes, which made exhausted Parisians walk for miles at night. However, there was still no enthusiasm for remote working. No doubt, the technology was still in its infancy, not yet democratized. The general public was probably not sufficiently aware of how to deal with complex and frequent technical problems on its own. The unions also played a role in slowing down the process, for fear of seeing their audience spread and their influence diminish. Business leaders feared for the confidentiality of their strategic data. They feared losing control of their teams’ activities. Middle management tried to preserve its visible perimeter through teams whose numbers were a measure of power. Employees, for their part, were afraid of being distanced from the decision-making centers. In addition to this diagnosis of the causes, working conditions at home did not always appear to be compatible with the requirements of companies.

So, why is there a development of remote working today?

First of all, let us not be too optimistic before going further. The probability that the whole ecosystem will tend to revert to the previous situation and ultimately slow down the development of remote work, that is, return to the “before” which seems ultimately more reassuring, because it is well known, is not zero. Nevertheless, let us try to list the factors that could, with the help of the generalized, conclusive and in situ experience of lockdown, give hope for real change.

The command of new technologies by individuals appears to be greater than that of their companies, which is a first factor.

Let us take the example of Microsoft Office. Very large organizations sometimes take several months, or even years, to roll out a new software version to all their employees, to the point where the last installed users benefit from the evolution when the next version is released. The first installers, on the other hand, often have to wait until the full rollout is complete before they can use their new version, due to internal compatibility issues. None of this happens in the home. The generalization of applications (apps), which are free or almost free, and software as a service (SaaS), where the service is accessed remotely instead of being installed on the user's own computer, has changed the technical landscape and usage. As soon as an application is released, it is acclaimed on social networks and in forums, tutorials flourish on YouTube and there are many sites for downloading apps. This is the case with Slack, Zoom and now Notion, to mention only the remote collective management tools. Users know how to combine classic software with very specific apps, how to work in external networks and how to find useful information wherever it is, including outside their company's databases.

The author of this text has personally experienced a caricatured situation in connection with the leading company in printing. When I asked a question to their hotline, I was told: "Go and look on the forums, you should find your answer. If not, call me back and I'll see what I can do!" Of course, this exchange took place a few years ago, when it was still possible to talk to a real person rather than chat (exchange via instant text messages, or supposedly so).

It is also known that online gaming has taught users to collaborate beyond the walls of their companies. Platforms such as Amazon have allowed them to start businesses with a few clicks and almost no investment. Forums have triggered a mechanism unknown 20 years ago: the search for solutions in communities of strangers who are trusted through rating systems.

It is from these developments that the possibility of immediate and painless implementation of "large-scale" remote working to cope with the Covid-19 pandemic was born.

3.2. Findings following lockdown

There are a number of observations that should be drawn from the experience of "full-scale remote working" that lockdown has allowed. The following are the findings that appear to be relevant at this stage.

Firstly, setting up and having all employees work remotely is not only possible, but also efficient and effective. Apart from a few organizations with plans, most of those who have implemented a good remote working solution have done so with the technical aspects in mind first. It is unlikely that these organizations did any dress rehearsal. Nor are they likely to have built, or maintained, a ready-made solution just in case. It was possible, in just a few days and based on the special knowledge of a few, to generalize what was done in a hurry. However, the lack of response to these implementations seems to show that things went rather well. However, the question of training for these new uses, for this new organization of work, could not be dealt with in a simple and serene manner.

Secondly, working remotely for a company is possible, and even comfortable in many cases. This is an additional motivation to make the transition from lockdown while keeping this possibility of organizing our professional activity in this way for at least a few days a week. It should be remembered that several studies have concluded that remote working is ideal, provided that it is limited to a maximum of one or two days per week. This limit is now being exceeded, with bank employees working in complete security, with all their software tools accessible from home. It seems that many employees, in the private sector as well as in the public sector, claim to work better and more under these conditions. The reduction of meeting times is also favored by remote workers. The exchanges on social networks, to be validated, show that many would be willing to work at home for the most part.

Many companies will use the experience of lockdown to rethink their infrastructure and organization, as well as to position themselves on other geographical markets at lower cost. For example, the emergence of a remote meeting solution such as Zoom shows that it is possible to make significant savings on travel time, on remote working equipment and on real-estate costs. Mid-sized companies, which often face capacity problems due to rapid growth, are likely to rethink their future relocations. Their 2.0 culture predisposes them to break with the logic of "all at the same time and in the same place".

Several companies, including world leaders such as Facebook and Twitter, have already announced that they will extend their remote working mode for many more months or even permanently. They expect to recruit from anywhere, as well as free themselves from the constraints of housing all their employees in expensive and geographically constraining proprietary spaces. The combination of platforms and remote working will form an extension of "uberized" tasks to intellectual services. This is what Amazon's "Mechanical Turk" solution prefigured, which made it possible to entrust parcels of work to service providers scattered all over the world for extremely low costs. This has the advantage of fragmenting tasks and therefore reducing the risk of hacking into a project or development.

The Covid-19 crisis has also shown that, when faced with a critical situation, companies were able to drastically shorten their decision-making processes, as well as break years of taboos on certain subjects. In particular, remote working was suddenly seen as a lucid and pragmatic issue. As the aftermath of the SARS-CoV-2 pandemic could continue for several months or even years, and some experts believe that other similar crises could follow, the use of remote working may become almost permanent. In fact, the inclusion of remote working in the practices of many European countries, led by Germany, is one of the explanations for better control of the epidemic. The right of withdrawal, the legal actions to demand the shutdown of an Amazon logistics platform in order to "improve the health protection of employees", will undoubtedly also accentuate the desire of company managers to reduce the weight of human error in their processes. Finally, it may be noted that, as has been the case for the last 25 years, the trade unions are rather inaudible on the subject of remote working, which means that they are likely to be relatively excluded from the organization of its development.

3.3. Foreseeable developments

We can now consider how the form of remote working, or more precisely its forms, will evolve in the years to come by first considering the weakening of the notion of enterprise that may result from such a development of work.

3.3.1. *Fragile nature of the concept of enterprise*

Many large groups have changed their name, country of incorporation, shareholding and sector of activity (e.g. La Générale des Eaux, which has become both Vivendi (telecoms, media) and Veolia (environment)). These radical and sometimes brutal changes call into question the *affectio societatis*, the special relationship between an employee and their employer. So do the frequent restructurings throughout the world. In these contexts, employees can feel that their role is fragile and that it can be called into question at any time. The collective project that is supposed to be the basis of a company's value is fading and employees feel that they must rely more on themselves to guarantee their future. This is undoubtedly the reason why business creation, supported by the self-entrepreneur status, motivated by the success stories of certain start-ups, is doing so well, despite the risks it entails.

The spin-offs of large groups, which separate themselves from activities deemed to be outside their core business, the aggregation of start-ups, cultivate this idea that autonomy is possible, positive and rewarding. The unemployment cover that has just been offered to company directors may play a decisive role in this development.

3.3.2. *Development of mixed statuses (self-employed employees)*

Possible for a long time, this dual activity, self-employed employee, is an option that should develop for the benefit of both parties:

– for the employee, it is a kind of safety net, a guaranteed income enabling them to start up and be able to take risks;

– for the company, it is the means for free initiative, creativity, enabling it to serve efficient resources and to gain in flexibility.

It is more than likely that the lockdown period will have been put to good use by those who were tempted by the experience of starting a business. It will be interesting to consult the statistics on business creation in 2020.

3.3.3. *Generalized multi-employment*

How many small business owners have given up on the idea of hiring executives for assignments that do not justify full-time work? How many executives have given up on taking advantage of 100% of their skills when faced with the obstacles of creating a consulting structure?

The use of multi-employer arrangements should become more widespread. In fact, selling one's skills as a financial analyst to two SMEs does not mean that one wants to start a business. Remote working will allow people with specialized skills, for which there is no sufficient demand in their region, to work for one, two or more companies, potentially geographically very far away.

Until now, collaborative work solutions did not offer conditions close enough to those of a physical meeting. Moreover, habits were hard to break. The "client" often felt that traveling to a one-hour meeting, even if the travel time was longer, was a sign of respect, or even subordination.

Lockdown, and the prospect of it happening again, will force the various economic players to reconsider remote working solutions. The value of a service will no longer be evaluated according to the time it has taken, but according to the contribution to the client structure's added value.

The generalization of evaluations and the principle of rating, long feared and contested, will also encourage the emergence of platforms for professional relations. Individuals will be invited to present and offer their skills, accepting that they will then be evaluated, as is now the case for doctor's consultations, mutual insurance company services or taxi fares.

3.3.4. *Development of globalized employment platforms*

While for the moment, Google, Apple, Facebook and Amazon (GAFA) have not investigated the field of employment, Amazon has already enabled the creation of 3 million merchants on its marketplace in 2019 (2 million in

2015). As many of these merchants are quasi-individuals who have a few products to sell but do not wish to take on the creation of an entrepreneurial structure, we can think that this practice is similar to a self-employment activity.

The same is true of the many online auction sites (e.g. Catawiki), which allow individuals to sell all kinds of items under excellent conditions. Le Bon Coin is another example of a platform that promotes the sale of products or services on a broad global scale. These activities are not included in national employment statistics, but they should be.

Of course, Uber, Deliveroo and AirBnB are nothing more than platforms for managing commercial activities. You only have to see how many attempts there are to have these activities, deemed independent, assimilated to salaried jobs to understand that if labor laws were to evolve towards greater flexibility and simplification (at least, as far as France is concerned), there would be a huge source of jobs in the service sector. Indeed, all these platforms today concern geolocalized activities that are impossible to relocate.

In the future, all intellectual services will be relocated and borders will no longer offer any protection. The openness that this practice will allow will offer a considerable source of employment.

3.4. Obstacles to the widespread development of remote working

As we have seen, even the extreme strikes of the Parisian transport system in the middle of winter did not see the remote working approaches put in place at the time. A leopard cannot change its spots! This is called resistance to change, and it is undoubtedly what has prevented the development of this solution, which so many employees are calling for. Of course, technologies have evolved considerably, both in terms of performance (upwards) and price (downwards), and the average skill level of employees in this area is in no way comparable.

However, we still tend to believe that what has become natural to us will quickly become the norm. There are a number of factors which are too often overlooked as obstacles to the development of remote working:

1) The equipment rate of households is not 100%, in terms of computers or printers.

Therefore, companies need to provide the right equipment, capable of sufficient performance. This is especially true since the software solutions implemented in companies are often cumbersome and sometimes complex. User support remains a sensitive issue, especially if employees want to work late at night or at the weekend from home.

Backup procedures must also be thought out in terms of these schedules, which have become free for users.

2) Working conditions at home are not always suitable.

While the level of facilities has increased, the same cannot be said of the size of the accommodation in the city. Being able to isolate ourselves to talk to colleagues or clients is not always possible, and these disparities in space can be a kind of discrimination, at a time when remote working is seen as an advantage.

3) Employee unions tend to oppose remote working, which makes worker mobilization more difficult and protests invisible.

4) Business leaders still fear the loss of sensitive data, as employees' personal workstations can be points of weakness in security systems.

5) Employees may fear isolation: losing the close link with the hierarchy, being informed only by what is made available, that is, no longer being able to grasp what is unofficial, means running the risk of being left out of opportunities. However, isolation also means technological vulnerability for those who do not master the tools to be used very well. This leads to the next point.

6) Companies must rethink their organization. This is not just a matter of deploying technical solutions and securing them. It is not enough to move existing solutions; they must also be rethought as building blocks for a new form of enterprise.

Employees will decide on their working hours, and this freedom must be made possible. Exchanges will be more structured, more written, less spoken. More prepared and less casual. The company's knowledge will have to be recorded, classified, updated, available and protected.

The hierarchical relationships will also have to be rethought, and relationship between performance and time worked on as well. New practices for measuring activity will have to be put in place, and for many companies, this will be counter-intuitive or even counter-cultural. The management function will inevitably be very different. What can be managed will be more limited and more automated. We should therefore see a net decrease in the number of managers. Tomorrow's managers will be facilitators and screen-based controllers. At the same time, we should see the development of horizontal mutual aid, but also self-training.

Companies that have structured their knowledge will use this data to build and distribute continuous online training, with assistance, coaching, tutorials, etc. All these approaches, which are still in their infancy, will now find an obvious use. What was until now the prerogative of large organizations will spread to smaller companies.

7) Remote working organizations will be based on relationships of trust, which is one of the essential keys to successful and sustainable remote working. This relationship of trust will either be reciprocal, or it will not exist at all.

In French engineering companies, quality control has become an indisputable practice in quality processes. However, in terms of customer service, for example, the work of yours truly with several social science research laboratories (carried out over five years) has shown that the higher the level of control, the lower the quality of service provided (2012–2016 Teletech International Study).

Ensuring that controls are reduced is a prerequisite for a successful remote working organization. However, many companies are still completely hostile to the idea. Looking "over the shoulder" of the employee, while affirming trust, is a reflex that will lead to failure.

8) What emerges from the feedback from neo-remote workers (in banking, for example) is the pleasure of working better. The fact that they

are able to harmonize their private and professional time more closely is a major advantage for them. The fact of being able to harmonize our private and professional time in a more refined way is a point often emphasized. The major paradigm shift, being judged on results and no longer on time spent, necessarily impacts the employee's feelings. This will underline the quality of the services provided and will render obsolete the procedures for controlling arrival and departure times, breaks, etc.

Meetings will be planned and recorded so that they can be shared with those who cannot attend. This will naturally lead to measuring the interest: how much time, compared to the time worked alone? How much time per department, per theme? What is known as "meetingitis", and which is so criticized in companies by employees who feel they are wasting their time, should be reduced in favor of more structured, better prepared and more exploited exchanges.

Remote working will also distribute among employees many of the tasks that are usually inherent in concentrating in one place of work: equipment, maintenance, catering, health, safety and working conditions, committee meetings, etc. The heaviness, the lack of agility of growing companies, will be lightened in favor of a voluntary contribution from users. Everyone will be responsible for cleaning their workstations and for their own catering, lighting, insurance, etc. All these elements will, paradoxically, accentuate the pleasure of working, thanks to this new feeling of freedom of action, autonomy and responsibility.

9) Resistance to change. Whatever the benefits expected by some or by others, the spectacular technological changes, the lockdowns in progress and perhaps to come, let us hold for certain that our resistance to change will do miracles… so that nothing changes!

It is with a wish that I would like to close this contribution: that we overcome all these obstacles and choose the path of fulfilment, creativity, freedom and co-construction. This opportunity that is offered to all of us, I mean to all human beings with all their differences, at the same time, this opportunity to reorient our lives and its links. This opportunity must be seized, because it may not come again soon.

3.5. References

Aguilera, A., Lethiais, V., Rallet, A., Proulhac, L. (2016). Le télétravail, un objet sans désir? *Revue d'Économie Régionale & Urbaine*, 1(1), 245–266 [Online]. Available at: https://doi.org/10.3917/reru.161.0245.

Centre d'analyse stratégique (2009). Le développement du télétravail dans la société numérique de demain. Report submitted to the Prime Minister, November.

Chicheportiche, O. (2012). Emploi dans les hotlines, que les opérateurs arrêtent de nous faire pleurer. *Teletech*, 18 September [Online]. Available at: https://www.zdnet.fr/actualites/emmanuel-mignot-teletech-emploi-dans-les-hotlines-que-les-operateurs-arretent-de-nous-faire-pleurer-39782583.htm.

Denis, D. (2011). Dynamiser le télétravail: Un enjeu décisif pour la croissance et l'emploi. Report of the Paris Chamber of Commerce and Industry.

Jacqunet, M. (2009). En Contact. May [Online]. Available at: https://en-contact.com/une-autre-pratique-du-metier-d%E2%80%99outsourceur-est-possible-teletech-l%E2%80%99a-demontre/.

Pontier, M. (2014). Télétravail indépendant ou télétravail salarié: Quelles modalités de contrôle et quel degré d'autonomie. *La Revue des Sciences de Gestion*, 1(1), 31–39 [Online]. Available at: https://doi.org/10.3917/rsg.265.0031.

4

The Digital Revolution and Religious Fact in the Context of Lockdowns Linked to the Coronavirus

4.1. Introduction

The acceleration of the transformations brought about by digital technology is profoundly disrupting society and the established economic models. Algorithms, big data, virtual reality, machine learning, robotics, artificial intelligence, connected objects, connected medicine, smart cities, blockchain, fintech (financial technology), increased use of the collaborative economy, the sharing economy, etc. – no part of life, no economic activity seems to escape the digital economy. Of course, spiritual life and the religious fact within our societies are not immune to the profound transformations brought about by the digital revolution. Over the past 30 years, the Internet has become an essential means of communication for all religions and their practice, particularly by contributing to enriching and renewing the community life of believers, which today can be estimated at several billion individuals.

The current pandemic, resulting from the coronavirus, has led the public authorities of most countries in the world to temporarily impose a lockdown (more or less strict) with profound repercussions on the personal (thus spiritual), family, social and economic lives of populations. The main objective of this chapter is to analyze the impact of lockdown on the spiritual lives of believers and the innovative contribution of digital tools for the

---

Chapter written by Éric FOGARASSY and François DEMONGEOT.

maintenance and renewal of religious practices within communities, subject to strong restrictions of individual and collective freedoms imposed by the public authorities. It is also an opportunity to question, on the "day after", the lessons to be learned from the greatest collective crisis that our humanity has had to face since the advent of the digital revolution, a crisis that affects all spheres of life, and in particular spiritual life and religion.

4.2. The lockdown concept

DEFINITION.– Lockdown is the act of confining someone or something, of locking them up in a restricted area, as well as the result of this action. By extension, "lockdown" is a safety procedure whose objective is to protect people or a population by isolating them in closed spaces.

Let us recall that the etymological origin of the word "confinement" or rather, lockdown, comes from the Latin *confinis*, meaning: that which confines, that which is contiguous, neighboring, that which touches, which is close to, which has the same limit. It is composed of *cum*: with; and *finis*: limit, border.

It should also be noted that this can be imposed or voluntary. Examples include persecuted religious communities, ghettos, prison life, maritime life, space travel and many other situations. The concept of containment has been of great interest to philosophers and has been the subject of a great deal of literature. In this regard, we can quote what Pascal wrote in his *Pensées*: "All the misfortune of men is that they do not know how to rest in a room." In the same spirit, I invite readers to read or reread Xavier de Maistre's *A Voyage Around My Room* (1795), a book devoted to the joys of confinement. Finally, let us not forget the famous novel *Robinson Crusoe* by Daniel Defoe (1719), which had a great literary success in the 18th century throughout Europe.

Can the situation of confinement experienced today be a source of enrichment and intellectual creation? Yes, if we refer to the history of our societies. Let us recall that it was during the Black Death epidemic in London (1655–1656) that the young Isaac Newton, forced to remain confined to his home, conceived the law of universal gravitation.

In the situation of lockdown imposed today by the pandemic, the four spheres of life identified, personal (including the spiritual dimension), family, social and professional, are configured differently. The "spheres of life" model (Table 4.1) is traditionally used to measure the gap between real life and desired life. By putting it back into the context of imposed confinement, it appears very relevant indeed: the coronavirus wizard has modified the respective sizes of the spheres, increasing the shares of the family and personal spheres, which include spirituality, and bringing them considerably closer together, even superimposing them, which is the exact effect of the digital tools that are becoming the indispensable auxiliary of work, entertainment and reflection. On the other hand, the social sphere has been considerably reduced, which is in fact the desired effect of lockdown, reducing the famous "R0" number (basic reproduction rate of a disease) and our social interactions.

4.3. Religions and religious facts

Religion is the set of beliefs, feelings, dogmas and practices that define the relationship of human beings with the sacred or a deity. A particular religion is defined by the elements specific to a community of believers: dogmas, sacred books, rituals, worship, sacraments, moral prescriptions, prohibitions, organization, etc. Most religions have developed from a revelation based on the exemplary history of a people, a prophet or a sage who taught an ideal of life.

Religion can be defined by its three main characteristics:

– religious beliefs and practices;

– religious feeling or faith;

– the union in the same community of those who share the same faith: the Church. This is what differentiates a religion from magic.

The study of religions, extinct or existing, shows the universal character of this phenomenon and a great variety in doctrines and ritual practices. A distinction is generally made between so-called primitive or animist religions, Eastern religions (Hinduism, Buddhism, Shintoism, Confucianism, Taoism, etc.) and the monotheistic religions derived from the Bible (Judaism, Christianity) and the Koran (Islam), Christianity having itself given rise to several Christian religions or churches (Catholic, Orthodox, Protestant, Evangelical, etc.).

A religious fact is a social fact like any other, a fact of religion, of the sacred.

For Jean-Paul Willaime, a specialist in religious sciences at the *École pratique des hautes études* (EPHE):

> The expression "religious facts" aims to grasp religious phenomena as "historical facts" on the one hand, and as "social facts" on the other, which is a way of emphasizing that religious phenomena are constructed as "facts" through various disciplinary approaches: historical, sociological, anthropological. This is not a challenge, but a way of qualifying, in the French language, the scientific approaches to religious phenomena (Willaime 2010).

4.4. The confinement concept and religious practices

The concept of confinement (imposed or voluntary) in the religious sphere has been closely linked to the history of religious practices since the beginning. The digital revolution and its tools (the Internet, social networks) have radically transformed, over the last 30 years, social links and practices within religious communities, particularly in the period of lockdown experienced during the Covid-19 pandemic.

Forms of confinement	
Confinement imposed on religious communities	***Voluntary confinement***
Persecuted religious communities	Religious sects
The Jewish sect of the Essenes	Monastic life (Carmel: a contemplative Catholic religious order)
Christianity in the catacombs (Roman Empire)	Life in a hermitage
Underground Christian communities in Cappadocia in the Middle Ages	Pilgrimages
The history of Jewish converts (Marranos) in Spain	
Protestant communities in France (revocation of the Edict of Nantes)	
Jewish ghettos	
Religious communities in the communist world (USSR, China, etc.)	

Table 4.1. *Types of confinement*

Since the origins of our societies, religions have integrated the concept of confinement (imposed or voluntary) as one of their structuring practices of functioning and development.

4.5. Religions in the face of great historical epidemics

As Catholics in 2020 celebrated an unprecedented Holy Thursday without rituals, and a Good Friday without the Stations of the Cross, Nicolas Balzamo, a historian at the University of Neuchâtel (Switzerland) and a specialist in religious history, explains how the Church has adapted to the great epidemics over the centuries (Balzamo 2020).

How did the Church organize itself to protect its faithful during the great epidemics?

The first knowledge of the mechanisms of contagion dates from the 19th century. Before that, the idea that gathering worshippers in a closed place was tantamount to opening the door to disease did not exist. At the time of the Great Plague (1348–1352), or the Black Death, there was even a resurgence of worship. Numerous religious events and processions were organized to ward off the plague. The first measures began to appear during the Renaissance, as when Archbishop Ambrose of Moscow decided in 1771, in the midst of the plague epidemic that hit Russia, to suppress a great collective prayer that was to be made before a famous icon. There was a riot; the archbishop was even killed.

In Europe, during the Spanish flu epidemic in 1918–1919, when the mechanisms of contagion were already well known, France severely restricted religious services. However, in the very pious Swiss canton of Valais, the priests refused the request of the civil authorities to celebrate masses in the open air instead, and gathered the faithful in their churches.

4.6. Impact of the digital revolution on religions and their practices

A drawing by the cartoonist Large published in the daily newspaper *Sud-Ouest* on April 4, 2020[1], sums up in a humorous way what is at stake in the debate.

1 Available at: https://www.sudouest.fr/.

Digital tools are an integral part of life in our modern societies and therefore impact all four spheres of life, including in particular the spiritual and religious sphere.

Stephen O'Leary, an American scholar of religion and communication and one of the first to analyze the role of new media in religious communities, argues that the advent of the Internet has been as revolutionary for the development of religions and their dissemination as the invention of the printing press (O'Leary 1996). Rosalind Hackett has written:

> The Internet is perhaps most associated with its ability to allow individuals to communicate with each other and connect to ever-widening networks of mutual interest. Interestingly, unconventional and even persecuted groups, such as Wiccans and neo-pagans in the United States, were among the first to take advantage of the Internet (Arthur). For some members, connecting through cyberspace would be comparable to the ritual of communion through "nature's energy" – which is central to pagan traditions. Recent research by Heidi Campbell on some Christian organizations has revealed that people who join online communities are looking for a sense of belonging, and want to unite in "the body of Christ" and not just get information (Campbell). For the millions of people who participate in chat rooms and belong to discussion forums, hasn't Yahoo become a new representation of Yahweh? (Hackett 2005)

Many scholars, however, question the nature of virtual communication: does it merely provide an "illusion of sociability" or does it demonstrate the existence of genuine online social interaction that can create and even strengthen bonds between communities of human beings in the offline world? Given that this notion of community is central to many religious traditions, this is an ongoing debate.

As a new interface for the exposure of religious beliefs, ritual and ethical practices, and as a site of community building and individuality, the Internet disrupts and reshapes not only these categories but many others as well, such as "world religion" and "minority religious groups". In other words, it is no longer necessary to set up a large-scale operation to reach (or be reached) globally. One rabbi remarked to a journalist that "for the first time in 2000 years, thanks to the Internet, Jewish ideas and values are interacting on an equal footing with other religions… There is a democratization of religion".

Until the middle of the 20th century, religious practices within confined communities could be summed up as living their faith "alone together", because they could no longer join their spiritual *community*, resulting in an extreme feeling of isolation and abandonment.

After World War II, the first religious broadcasts on radio and television (the "Mass at home") were set up.

Thirty years ago, the Web and its digital revolution were born. Thanks to the "grace" of the Internet and social networks, we can continue to share our hope and faith within our religious community, in many situations of distance or isolation, such as confinement.

Today, addressing God through our cell phone is what many mobile applications offer. All religions have launched into e-spirituality, a new way of praying or meditating that is by no means ephemeral. The number of mobile applications related to religion, as well as to secular meditation, is growing rapidly. This phenomenon may come as a surprise, given that digital tools embody our consumer society, the zapping from one task to another and therefore the distance from a form of intimacy with the sacred or with ourselves. Yet, "the movement gained momentum from 2008 onwards in Anglo-Saxon religions", says Christophe Deshayes, author of a study on the theme of living well thanks to digital technology (Deshayes 2013). "They wanted to develop the communitarian side and protect their children from the Internet by creating their own tools". Since then, all religions have created apps that meet the needs of their followers. "Regarding Judaism and Islam, the applications are mainly used to recall the rules and help with their interpretation", says David Douyère (Douyère and Antoine 2018), Professor of Information and Communication Sciences at the University of Tours and specialist in religions. "This is logical for these religions that have maintained ritual obligations that the faithful must follow in their daily lives. Among Christians, the applications are more oriented towards prayer."

Far from an ephemeral fashion movement, these digital tools are in fact part of a form of tradition. "Apps play the role of the images of piety that appeared in the 14th century" (Douyère and Antoine 2018). They have two characteristics in common: they are portable and they are intimate, since the phone contains our entire life. Indeed, religions have always needed a material anchor, which has changed as technology has evolved, and when it comes to new technologies, "the churches have never been behind", says Jonveaux. They give the impression of being archaic, but in fact they were very quick to use the printing press, television, etc.

Today, mobile applications are clearly a sign of modernity. At the Eucharistic Youth Movement (EYM), promoting *Click To Pray*, the official app of the Pope's Global Prayer Network, was an obvious choice. "We have no choice if we want the younger generation to feel involved", says Marion de Marcellus, former director of the EYM.

Religious institutions have other motivations: to bring the faithful back to the congregation at a time when true digital churches are appearing, to animate a community, social networks and applications are particularly suitable tools at a time when churches are being deserted and priests are aging. "Applications have the great merit of making a community visible", insists David Douyère. *Click To Pray* displays the number of people praying at the same time in black and white. However the element that most drives institutions to invest in the Apple and Android stores is undoubtedly the desire for evangelization.

4.7. Main digital tools used during the Covid-19 pandemic

The tools most used during the Covid-19 lockdown were ultimately quite similar in both the professional and private spheres. An analysis made of the most downloaded applications during the lockdown (Smaïl 2020) highlighted the following:

– *Discord*: a remote video conferencing application that initially targeted the online gaming and e-sports communities.

– *Zoom Meetings*: online conferencing application, used in the professional and associative world to organize remote meetings.

– *Houseparty*: application to organize meetings between friends; it informs you when your friends or contacts are available to chat.

– *Plato*: group game application; its success is mainly due to its social character and the possibility of playing with friends and family.

– *WhatsApp*: a safe bet for online messaging that replaces SMS and allows, in addition to messages, video calls to be made and audio and video messages to be shared.

– *Spiral Roll*: puzzle game application.

– *TikTok*: a social music network application popular with teenagers.

– *Microsoft Teams*: application used by many companies for daily communication.

In France, over the period from March 16–22, 2020, these applications were downloaded between 185,000 times, for the first, Discord, and 65,000 times, for the last, Microsoft Teams.

All these applications, even the game ones, are characterized by a high level of interaction. Pascal was right, humanity seeks above all entertainment, and entertainment in society.

4.8. Adapting religious practices during lockdown for the coronavirus crisis

The current pandemic has led the public authorities to ban all religious ceremonies that usually take place in all places of worship: churches, synagogues and mosques. Thus, the coronavirus profoundly disrupted the ritual practices of the Easter week among Christians. The supreme authorities of the Catholic Church drew from the consequences of the world pandemic by publishing new decrees specifying the measures to be taken so that celebrations from Holy Thursday to Easter Day could be held in the absence of the faithful. The priests were allowed, exceptionally, to celebrate Mass in an appropriate place without the participation of the people. Some ritual acts changed: the washing of the feet, which was already optional, was omitted, as was the procession following the Mass of the Lord's Supper. The act of adoration of the cross by kissing was limited to the celebrant alone, the Easter vigil was celebrated exclusively in cathedrals and parish churches and Easter communion, with bread and wine, was reserved for the celebrant and was subject to health precautions. The same restrictions were imposed on Protestant communities. As far as the Jewish community was concerned, the traditional meal (the Seder) on the occasion of Pesach (Jewish Passover) was also adapted to the situation at the time. For the same reasons, the Muslim holidays of Ramadan were subject to the same restrictions. Finally, we should note the suppression of major religious pilgrimages involving millions of pilgrims (Lourdes, Mecca, Jerusalem, etc.).

4.8.1. *Christian worship*

Catholic and Protestant worship has taken many initiatives through adaptation, reinvention or creation. Among these are:

– the televising of religious celebrations; the oldest program (*Le jour du Seigneur*, on France 2), never interrupted since 1947, has seen its audience increase strongly (triple) Sunday after Sunday, despite (or thanks to) the very sober character of the celebrations (Barba 2020), alongside numerous retransmissions, in particular during Holy Week on KTO, and even on France 3 Alsace on Good Friday for an ecumenical prayer, which had never been done before (Gramond 2020);

– the communication tools set up by the dioceses, such as that of Alsace, with regular messages from the authorities, spiritual proposals, encouragement to give and a course of rediscovery of the texts of the Bible (Alsace catholique 2020);

– the reinforced communication of the major actors in charity and solidarity, such as Caritas, on social networks and traditional radio stations, and the implementation of special initiatives for the most deprived (Fondation Caritas France 2020);

– proposals for remote pilgrimages encouraged by the dioceses (Église catholique 2020a);

– tools for preparing for remote sacrament, such as a virtual marriage preparation course offered by the CPM movement (Centre de préparation au mariage);

– proposals to replace pilgrimage trips with virtual ones, as the specialized agency Ictus Voyages[2] has done.

Given the profusion of initiatives on the Internet and social networks, are there not new forms of community practices to be highlighted, especially among Catholics?

2 For more information, see https://www.ictusvoyages.com.

On this question, Sophie de Villeneuve collected for the newspaper *La Croix* the point of view of Benoist de Sinety, the vicar general of the diocese of Paris. He states that:

> The establishment of celebrations relayed by the Internet is necessary because it makes the absence less painful, but it is not sufficient. I would say that it is a stopgap. This is a question that has been asked since the Second Vatican Council, which, by recalling that the Eucharist is the source and summit of the Church, may have led us to think that without the Mass, no Church is possible, no Christian life is possible, no Gospel is possible. This deserves to be qualified. One of the great merits of the impossibility of believers gathering in church is that it could lead to the emergence of the family liturgy, a form of celebration which French Catholics are not at all used to. The Jews have always had it. The Protestants have always done it, to some extent. The Orthodox practiced family liturgies under the communist regime, which forbade them any public celebration (de Villeneuve 2020).

Finally, let us note that many religious are already pointing out the limits of digital technology, wishing to resist the temptation to disembody pastoral care (the art of living together in reference to Jesus Christ) in a world that is already finding it increasingly difficult to distinguish the virtual from the real.

4.8.2. *Jewish worship*

In Israel, where all places of worship have been closed, regardless of religion, there was a debate among rabbis as to whether it was possible to use a video conferencing application to allow the family to meet in another way. Some rabbis felt that “in an emergency situation”, it was possible to use such applications to celebrate the holiday with “elderly or sick people”. The Chief Rabbinate of Israel was opposed to this, as there was no question of “desecrating a holiday”.

4.8.3. *Muslim worship*

In France, all mosques have been closed following the appeal launched on March 15, 2020 by the French Council of the Muslim Faith (*Conseil français du culte musulman*, CFCM), an association whose mission is to represent the Muslim faith in France to the public authorities. For Ramadan, the holy month of fasting and one of the five pillars of Islam, which began on April 24, the CFCM maintained its instruction and "encouraged the faithful to perform their daily prayers at home". Gatherings for prayers and meals to break the fast, traditionally organized by mosques and charities, were thus banned. On the other hand, the tradition of fasting was maintained. The CFCM also called on Muslim leaders and imams to "use all means at their disposal to ensure the continuity of the relationship with the faithful". Practitioners, confined to their homes, were invited to follow the preaching in the mosques via social networks or YouTube. In this context, the imams of the Great Mosque of Paris proposed a daily sermon on Radio Orient.

Nevertheless, lockdown is experienced as a constraint by all religious communities because the virtual community will never be a real community. Thus, for Christians, the sacrament has its full value only in the joint presence of concrete and real facts with spiritual help. Every sacrament is "the visible sign of an invisible grace". The water of baptism and the anointing of the sick are indispensable elements of the sacrament that technology cannot provide. Moreover, a life of faith is the meeting of a spiritual life and concrete acts. If the former can be enriched in times of confinement, the latter is impoverished in the same circumstances.

During lockdown, the need for concreteness and community of proximity was expressed, for example, by the simultaneous ringing of church bells throughout France on March 25 at 7:30 p.m. With this sign, the Church wanted to send a message of fraternity, as well as to allow the French to establish a concrete, audible link with the normal place of their religious practice, in this case, the parish. Indeed, the Church has always been organized in territorial communities, the parishes and not in the communities of elections that are those of the social networks. In the Christian community, there are no differences of social or geographical origin, but a community of brothers, as opposed to the communities of the social networks which are more often than not interiors. In the Christian Church, there are no longer Jews or Greeks, but Christians arc one in Christ, as St. Paul wrote in his letter to the Galatians in *The New Testament*.

The sacraments cannot be experienced, either in confinement or through technology. The first televised Masses (the world's first in France in 1947, with the midnight Mass at Christmas) gave rise to theological reflections and warnings from the episcopates, reminding us that they cannot replace the physical communion of the community, independently of the problem of Eucharistic communion. The Catholic Church insists that it is anthropologically wrong to consider that virtual reality is able to replace the real, tangible and concrete experience of the visible and historical Christian community, and the same is true for the sacraments and celebrations, as the Jesuit Antonio Spadaro has noted in a study on cyber-theology (Spadaro 2018).

On the other hand, during the lockdown period, the only ones allowed to exercise their "normal" spiritual activity were the hospital chaplains, who were able to accompany the dying in the place of the families, through their presence and prayer; but this was done under very constrained conditions and without being able to administer a sacrament (Vantighem 2020). The many funerals held in very small groups were also a source of suffering for many families, and at the end of the lockdown, many ceremonies will be organized to pray for the deceased and to support the mourning of relatives.

Exercising concrete charity ("To be Martha as well as Mary") is not possible by remaining confined. It should be noted that charitable organizations, such as Caritas, operate their reception and support services with many volunteers, most of whom are retired. The average age of the volunteers has led those in charge of the associations to ask them to stay at home and to ask for the help of young people, such as the scouts, to replace them in certain tasks. The Church has mobilized for the weakest, but the exercise of this charity requires not being confined (Église catholique 2020b).

The limits of lockdown for religious practice in places of worship (churches, mosques, synagogues) are obviously posed in similar terms for all religions. For example:

– the ritual of communion within the various Christian communities. Thus, the faithful receive a host from the priest (among Catholics), a piece of bread or sometimes a host from the pastor (among Protestants), or bread and wine from the priest (among Orthodox);

– the accompaniment of the deceased during funerals for all religions, which represents for anthropologists, since the origins of humanity, one of the foundations of the passage to civilization;

– the physical experience of pilgrimage, which represents an individual or group journey to a holy place for religious purposes in a spirit of devotion (for Christians, to the Vatican, Jerusalem, Lourdes and Santiago de Compostela; for Muslims, to Mecca; and for Jews, to the Wailing Wall in Jerusalem).

4.9. Digital revolution and religious practices: the future

We have seen how the digital revolution has supported religions and their practices for more than 30 years, and how it has contributed, during the exceptional period of lockdown, to maintaining and renewing in depth the spiritual life of religious communities, provided that the faithful have access to these new technologies. It is therefore not useless to wonder about the rate of penetration of digital tools in our societies, at the global level. Let us recall some recent figures on this subject: in 2019, the number of Internet users amounted to 4.38 billion, with an increase of 9% over one year (Séblain 2019). Thus, 57% of the world's population had the Internet and 45% were registered on social networks. These figures are to be compared with the estimated number of believers for the three major monotheistic religions. Today, there are an estimated 2.4 billion Christians in the world, 1.9 billion Muslims and 15 million Jews. It can be estimated that the proportion of believers equipped with the Internet is comparable to the figures published for the world population. We can therefore conclude that almost half of the believers confined at the global level, via the current pandemic, have not been able to take advantage of the digital revolution for their religious practices.

However, the digital revolution underway worldwide is expected to continue its unstoppable progress. This evolution will automatically lead to an increase in the number of Internet users wishing to access the services provided by digital technology for their religious practices (participation in worship and community life). The main populations concerned are naturally people who are alone, isolated, ill and elderly. In a more prospective way, the generalization of new digital tools, such as simultaneous translators, should contribute to bringing together religious communities, today unable to communicate orally because of language barriers. We can anticipate the growing role that digital tools will play in the communication, organization and management of large international charismatic and religious gatherings, such as the World Youth Day (WYD) or the pilgrimage to Mecca.

The lockdowns we have just experienced have made us aware of the extent to which digital technologies impact all spheres of our lives: personal, family, social and professional. The exceptional situation of lockdown has considerably increased the planetary needs in telecommunication tools. In this context, Big Tech (Google, Apple, Facebook, Amazon, Microsoft) have shown their ability to meet the global demand, each of them posting double-digit growths, both in terms of turnover and net profits. These major groups have also shown that they can innovate and adapt, at a moment's notice, to the demands of a global market in the midst of a health and economic crisis. Satya Nadella, the CEO of Microsoft, was able to write: "We have experienced two years of digital transformation in just two months" (Kerdellant 2020). In the end, society in all its dimensions, including the religious sphere and its practices, should benefit significantly from this ongoing technological revolution.

4.10. References

Alsace catholique (2020). 12e dimanche du temps ordinaire. *Alsace Catholique* [Online]. Available at: https://www.alsace.catholique.fr/les-services/service-formation/saveurs-devangile/375044-saveurs-devangile/.

Balzamo, N. (2020). De la peste noire au coronavirus: La religion catholique face aux épidémies. *GEO – Histoire*, 10 April

Barba, D. (2020). La messe en direct sur France 2: L'ascension des audiences en période de confinement. *France Inter* [Online]. Available at: https://www.franceinter.fr/emissions/capture-d-ecrans/capture-d-ecrans-10-avril-2020.

De Villeneuve, S. (2020). Une Église sans messe? *La Croix*, 25 April.

Deshayes, C. (2013). Un marché de grand avenir: Le bien-vivre grâce au numérique. *Journal de l'Ecole de Paris*, March/April.

Douyère, D. and Antoine, F. (2018). Penser l'entrelacs des religions et des médias. *Revue Française des Sciences de l'information et de la communication*, 13.

Église catholique (2020a). Confinement: Les pèlerinages virtuels ont la cote ! Église catholique en France [Online]. Available at: https://eglise.catholique.fr/sengager-dans-la-societe/sante/coronavirus-covid19/par-dela-le-confinement/par-dela-le-confinement-jeunes-chretiens-eglise/498467-confinement-pelerinages-virtuels/.

Église catholique (2020b). L'Église face au Coronavirus-Covid19. Foi, Espérance, charité: Par-delà le confinement. Église catholique en France [Online]. Available at: https://eglise.catholique.fr/sengager-dans-la-societe/sante/coronavirus-covid19/par-dela-le-confinement/.

Fondation Caritas France (2020). COVID19 – Confinés mais mobilisés – la Fondation Caritas France soutient Parcours d'Exil. Fondation Caritas France [Online]. Available at: https://www.fondationcaritasfrance.org/2020/04/confines-mais-mobilises-la-fondation-caritas-france-soutient-parcours-dexil/.

Gramond, F. (2020). REPLAY – Émission spéciale "Le temps du silence": Une célébration œcuménique du Vendredi saint. *France info* [Online]. Available at: https://france3-regions.francetvinfo.fr/grand-est/bas-rhin/strasbourg-0/replay-emission-speciale-temps-du-silence-celebration-oecumenique-du-vendredi-saint-1813306.html.

Hackett, R.I.J. (2005). Religion et Internet. *Diogène*, 211, 3.

Kéderllant, C. (2020). Les Gafam applaudissent le Covid-19. *L'usine nouvelle*, 3664 [Online]. Available at: https://www.usinenouvelle.com/editorial/les-gafam-applaudissent-le-covid-19.N975061.

O'Leary, S. (1996). Cyberspace as sacred space: Communicating religion on computer networks. *Journal of the American Academy*, LXIV(4).

Séblain, B. (2019). Digital, social media, mobile et e-commerce en 2019. *We Are Social* [Online]. Available at: https://wearesocial.com/fr/blog/2019/01/global-digital-report-2019.

Smaïl (2020). Covid-19: Liste des 10 applications mobile les plus téléchargées en France pendant le confinement. *EmarkerterZ* [Online]. Available at: https://www.emarketerz.fr/covid-19-liste-top-10-applications-telechargees-confinement/.

Spadaro, A. (2014). *Cyber théologie – Penser le christianisme à l'heure d'Internet.* Lessius – Éditions jésuites, Brussels.

Vantighem, V. (2020). Coronavirus: "On nous demande de prier à travers une vitre...". Le délicat travail des aumôniers. *20 Minutes* [Online]. Available at: https://www.20minutes.fr/societe/2755095-20200405-coronavirus-demande-prier-travers-vitre-delicat-travail-aumoniers.

Willaime, J.-P. (2010). Faits religieux. In *Dictionnaire des faits religieux*, Azria, R. and Hervieu-Léger, D. (eds). Presses universitaires de France, Paris.

5

Old and New Rituals Throughout the Covid-19 Pandemic

This chapter has been written in the wake of the pandemic. Thus, the deaths that plunged many regions and cities of the world into mourning, the concerns that surrounded the progress of the epidemic, the time for reflection that the lockdowns allowed, the funeral ceremonies, the media events and the political recollections that punctuated the long period of Covid-19 have brought back the role and practice of rituals.

People often behave in ways that, at first glance, are inexplicable or curious. These mysteries are usually rooted in an unconscious social memory. This is why psychology, sociology and communication sciences try to decipher these behaviors, to analyze them, to understand them. We will see below how rituals are places, hubs of communication and negotiation, but they are also sources of monetary exchange as soon as a ritual is tamed and transformed by the market system. This is true of death, which is one of the major elements of the pandemic that is still going on at the time of writing. With Covid-19, focusing on death becomes important, because this fact – which is in the realm of normality, given every human being is mortal – becomes an event that, as a consequence of the pandemic, is presented every evening by the announcement of the "daily death count" on television.

A theory known as affordance (a neologism derived from the verb *to afford*) was proposed by the sociologist Thierry Bardini following the psychologist James Gibson, who gave form to the concept of affordance in

---

Chapter written by Bruno SALGUES.

1977. Bardini's proposal consisted of analyzing the relationship between the object, in our case Covid-19, and its user. With affordance, it is a question of measuring "what the user gives to his object" through a combination of actions, content and events, including rituals (Bardini 1996). Thierry Bardini thus goes beyond the theory of inscription (which is the space for the confrontation of body and mind with death) put forward by the philosopher Maurizio Ferraris, through which each event of importance imposes an inscription.

5.1. The ritual notion

In order to be anchored in consciousness, the memory of humanity and of people needs to use the notion of an event to highlight salient facts and to refer to benchmarks, including rituals, as both valuable and easily discernible points of reference. One of the most significant ritual moments is that surrounding death, particularly following the progression of an epidemic, even though digital technology such as photography, film and video now allow us to "live after death".

The transhumanist movements have seized upon the particular ritual of death with a philosophical idea derived from religion, which is to establish immortality by making the most perfect copy of a human possible and to fight the idea of death. Previously, physicians' thinking on death was limited to ethical approaches, such as how to limit the number of people who are not cared for, and how to prevent euthanasia and genocide. More recently, ethical debates have focused on birth control, abortion and genetic manipulation.

5.1.1. *Religious and secular rituals*

DEFINITION.– In its primary sense, a ritual is the set of ceremonies of worship in use in a religious community or the actions and words prescribed by the liturgy of a religion.

Rituals are also key points in social life, and they play an important role in the staging of major life events (birth, marriage, graduation, death). In this regard, the relationship between death and religious ceremonies is well established. By analogy, collective social behaviors have been equated with religious rituals, within which repetition and sacred or symbolic elements are also present. On a broader level, certain secular social customs or habits, such as death notices in local newspapers, have been referred to as "rituals". The question that arises is how obituaries transform, disappear or are reborn in the digital age.

Although death is a fact that is not entirely linked to humanity, insofar as certain animals, such as chimpanzees, experience it, humanity is capable of creating it spontaneously in many circumstances. Robinson Crusoe marking the days on his desert island is the best known image of ritualization. This literary episode illustrates one of the characteristics of rituals, particularly through death, namely the fact of marking, inscribing or engraving the memory of the ritual event. The digital marking of death has replaced the engraving in marble that was previously intended to be immutable. This marking was highlighted in an emblematic way by the front page of the *New York Times* on May 24, 2020. A list of 1,000 names was published on this front page, along with short biographies of the deceased individuals, all victims of coronavirus and representing only 1% of the Covid-19-related deaths in the United States. A journalist from the French daily paper *Ouest-France* described this emblematic front page as "cold as a blade" (Ouest-France 2020).

Ritual practice always has sacred or symbolic aspects. Rituals, while based on real data related to the four elements (earth, fire, water, air), very often link them to supernatural or magical circumstances. This is the case during communion, which is part of the ritual of Catholic Mass. Indeed, the unleavened bread is seen as the body of Christ, and the wine his blood. The act of ingesting the bread and drinking the wine, as practiced by the priest during communion, is not considered anthropophagy. Rituals serve to distinguish the sacred from the lay or, more precisely, to bring the sacred into the lay domain, into collective life. Of the front-page story just mentioned, Marc Lacey, editor of the *New York Times*, said, "I wanted something that people could read back in 100 years to understand the weight of what we're going through". So, the notion of a "brand" is still very much alive in ritual gestures.

How is the ritual object, especially in the case of death, reified, chosen? How does the very real relationship between two people – modified by "distance" – become a "thing" to be analyzed as such? This notion of a brand or branding is very important in rituals. We will see later that in the literature, this reification takes place in different ways, notably through the image in the thinker McLuhan, the voice in Ferraris and the apparatus in the Italian philosopher Giorgio Agamben.

AGAMBEN'S DEFINITION OF THE APPARATUS.– "Anything that has, in one way or another, the capacity to capture, orient, determine, intercept, shape, control, and ensure the gestures, conducts, opinions, and discourses of living beings" (Agamben 2009).

5.1.2. *Function of ritual recognition*

Generally speaking, rituals have a recognition function and allow for integration into a group. Death is traditionally associated with a religion ("that which connects"). Rituals also take other forms, such as vocabulary or jargon (e.g. the legal jargon used by lawyers) or attire (white coats in a hospital). Ritual elements are embedded in a social reality. The evolution of societies and technological changes destroy certain rituals and recreate others. This notion of recognition is therefore more complex than that of branding mentioned above.

Digital technologies contribute to the acceleration of time. Health-related technologies lead to questioning the notion of death. The consequence is the rejection or contestation of all the acquired knowledge. Traditional rituals thus appear anachronistic. Past rituals are depreciated, as well as reinvented, particularly because of digital technologies, because human beings cannot live without them.

5.2. Decline of traditional rituals

5.2.1. *Causes of decline*

The decline of traditional rituals seems to be essentially a permanent human search for freedom from taboos and constraints, from everything that seems established, unchangeable and outdated in order to achieve greater individual freedom. Today's world is marked by the immediacy of the digital world. Such evolution has consequences in terms of understanding religious morality, which is perceived confusedly as a constraint of another age, with regard to married life, contraception, education and death. Thus, we can see today a parallel decline in the ritual value of religious ceremonies. The decline in certain religious practices is a reality that has an impact on societies in particular. Traditional religious ceremonies impose presence, whereas the digital world invites us to virtuality.

The second reason for the decline of rituals, including those related to death, is to be found in the questioning of the clear, precise, defined social role that the rituals conferred on each individual, through rites of passage. After an exam, we traditionally become a bachelor, and after a marriage, we become a couple. This social framing no longer corresponds to the current aspiration of individuals, which is characterized by the use of digital communication tools, including social networks. Through these tools, such as Facebook, Twitter or Snapchat, each individual can play several roles. An individual is therefore simultaneously an employee of a company, as well as a promoter of their sport and a member of an association defending a cause. The result is the breakdown of social groups that used to take care of the human being from birth to death. The disappearance of this previously important temporality contributes to the expiration of a whole series of rituals, including the ritual practices surrounding death.

Some rituals are therefore falling into disuse. There are two explanations for this:

– certain rituals have not been able to adapt to changes in the cultural and technological context;

– some rituals are no longer understood and the people performing the ritual are actually losing the sense of its deeper meaning.

The Catholic Church is confronted with this problem with regard to religious practices, particularly in the context of the funeral Mass, which can nevertheless be of great benefit to everyone if minimum reflection on symbolic rituals is carried out and if a critical spirit is involved.

Thus, the funeral Mass consists of four rituals[1]:

– the ritual of light, the lighted Paschal candle, symbolizing the presence of the risen Christ, whose light enlightens the world. The gesture of taking the flame of the Paschal candle to light the candles that surround the coffin signifies that the light of the risen Christ is the source of our hope in the

1 Translated definition based on the *Cybercuré* website, available at: https://cybercure.fr/je-prie/funerailles-obseques/article/celebration-of-obsequies-funerailles.

resurrection, and reminds us that the deceased became a child of God at their baptism;

– the ritual of the end or of the cross: this ritual is often represented by a cross, but it is not always practiced; it involves putting a cross on the coffin, or recalling its presence on the coffin, reminding us that Jesus loved us until he died for us;

– the ritual of incense, a sign of respect for the deceased symbolizing "the prayer that goes up to God";

– the ritual of sprinkling "holy water on the coffin, which recalls the water of baptism by which the Christian is immersed in the death of Christ, in order to rise with him".

It is easy to understand that these rituals cannot be easily digitalized, unless virtual reality or 3D holograms one day make it possible to implement them. On the other hand, it should be noted that these rituals can be found in the advice given by management coaches when they express the behavior to show towards colleagues.

As for the loss of influence of the village community, of the family, it erases all the rituals marking the stages of belonging to a community, the children no longer coming to spend their holidays in the family home where the grandparents live (see the novel *At God's Pleasure* by Jean d'Ormesson), the family dispersed across cities no longer meeting in full at communion, at the marriage of a cousin, a nephew, etc. Finally, the use of many rituals for political purposes has accentuated the phenomena of rejection, the refusal of ritual practice appearing to constitute an act of political resistance, for example, in Ettore Scola's film, *A Special Day*, the refusal to participate in a mass meeting, in this case the celebration of Mussolini and Hitler's fascism.

5.2.2. *Contradictory manifestations of the decline of rituals*

The manifestations of the decline of rituals seem to correspond either to a strong disaffection with them or to a superstitious attachment to them.

Marriage, which is often no longer achieved during a lifetime, thus loses its ritual value. It is clear that wedding ceremonies have been strongly affected by the epidemic.

The same is true for death, as life can now be extended – or is about to be – through transplants and bionic tools. Moreover, registration tools allow records to be made help to extend life. This is the promise of transhumanism. In fact, audio, then video recordings, and now holograms, make it possible to create a kind of virtual life.

On the other hand, some rituals give rise to almost superstitious forms of attachment. For some individuals, certain ritual practices must be continued absolutely, for fear of seeing them disappear forever. The Latin liturgy, advocated by the fundamentalist currents of the Catholic Church (e.g. the movement of Archbishop Lefèvre, the Priestly Fraternity of Saint Pius X, in the 1970s), is still present today on social networks.

5.3. Old rituals substituted by new ritual phenomena

Rituals are constantly being reinvented through technology. In contemporary society, there is a desire – sometimes rather clumsy – to create new rituals. Through technology, the actors of social networks are looking for marks of adherence to common values, as well as marks of re-birth and belonging to a specific community, which now go through a "like". These marks have a function of belonging to a "New World", in which the old reference points are more or less in ruins. Wanting to "like" death is a kind of challenge. As for dead people whose likes appear after their death, Facebook explains that old likes can "surface" if no one notifies the company of the account user's death.

> A Facebook spokesperson says "likes" of dead people can occur if an account is not "memorialized". If no one notifies Facebook that the account owner is dead, Facebook thus continues to operate, assuming the person is alive. In this case, a person's likes from months ago can still resurface in their friends' News Feeds, as Facebook recycles the likes long after they have occurred (El Hassani 2012).

5.3.1. *In social life*

In social life, new rituals linked to new forms of social life are taking the place of family ones. With Facebook, death is moving out of the family framework to a kind of extension to everyone.

Through clothing and body fashions, and through membership of this or that group (rockers, tattooed people, pierced people, etc.), ritual phenomena are recreated that are perhaps more ephemeral than traditional rituals, sacrificing themselves to the tastes of an era, but whose lively and sometimes very dynamic character cannot be denied. This notion of rituals of partnership cannot be overlooked, for they were numerous in the first wave of the Covid-19. We belonged to the community of caregivers because we applauded them by going out of our house at 8 p.m. during lockdown. Thus, the culture of the light blue-green coat appeared, on the one hand, in television images, as well as a color reference in cartoons, including those of the French press cartoonist and caricaturist Plantu. Some new rituals refer to a certain belonging. Thus, the rituals of social comfort, of success, extend beyond the framework of the main home and are multiplied in the practice of weekends and trips abroad. During the period of lockdown linked to Covid-19, it was rather the rituals of discomfort that emerged, such as of course the discomfort of being confined, as well as that of women and men with exposed professions, ranging from the medical profession to garbage collectors and public transport professions. Other practices aimed at an objective opposite to the desire to belong to a group, seeking to distinguish themselves from it. Thus, such and such an individual, an anonymous number of a large company, will strive to be known and recognized by others by practicing a sport in fashion, such as hang gliding or ultra-light aviation, thereby participating in a ritual sports practice allowing them to distinguish themselves from others.

5.3.2. *Rituals as an expression of a current of thought*

Modern rituals are the means of expression of certain currents of thought, of a certain protest (vegans, ecological demonstrations, hunger strikes, etc.), which is concentrated, with Covid-19, at the level of health professionals. Why question the new place of rituals? Because they are poorly known or poorly interpreted. The place of ritual phenomena in contemporary society seems to have been exacerbated by Covid-19, calling for specific new roles for the state, and therefore for political personnel.

To conclude this third point, it can be said that the reinvented rituals are alive, more mobile, more diversified and more contradictory than those that punctuated the lives of our ancestors. These rituals, which have changed form with the epidemic, must have a new place in society.

5.4. Poorly understood rituals

5.4.1. *Unknowingly engaging in rituals*

The rational, rationalist, Cartesian dominance of our industrial societies seems to favor laws and regulations to the detriment of rituals. However, the revival of ethnological analysis, no longer of primitive societies (Lévi-Strauss), but of our own societies, underlines the importance of ritual phenomena that we all practice without knowing it (Bourdieu).

In spite of everything, the temptation is strong for the politician, the trade unionist, the academic or the sociologist to place ritual practice in the domain of the irrational, outside the field of the social world. This would be a serious mistake, because today rituals are at the crossroads of all negotiations (rituals of union–management meetings, ritual elections and above all rituals of television news, like the six o'clock news).

5.4.2. *Dealing with the new place of rituals*

Certain rituals attempt to freeze societies: legal jargon, for example, renders trials incomprehensible; medical vocabulary renders the medical world esoteric and "magical"; the syntax of economics renders economic phenomena incomprehensible. In this case, rituals are an obstacle to communication and dialogue, and they freeze a "society" which, as a result, risks sinking into decadence.

Other rituals, on the other hand, remain the only remaining links between members of a community – increasingly global and less local – in which tasks are divided and fragmented, while converging towards a common goal.

5.4.3. *Protective role of the State*

Today's State must be secular, in the sense that it must not favor one ritual phenomenon over another (subsidizing classical music concerts is a common practice in this regard, unlike subsidizing pop concerts).

The State must show tolerance for the diversity of rituals, first of all by protecting the freedom of the press. The State must emphasize and take better account of all spontaneous social phenomena, but not manipulate them for political purposes, a practice that could appear as a return to fascism, a soft and well-meaning fascism.

5.5. Performative rituals

5.5.1. *Rituals and order*

Originally, the ritual describes that which is accomplished in accordance with order, according to the Sanskrit etymology of this word (*rita* = order). Humanity, subjected to the disorder of the human condition, engages in a movement that must lead them to overcome this condition to find harmony. Order is suggested to them by all of the ancestral and mythical messages, through proverbs and rituals. These rituals can have several different meanings and correspond either to rituals of protection, or to rituals of opposition or poor integration.

5.5.2. *Rituals of protection*

Society takes on the struggle against attempts to destroy social unity. It seeks a continual conversion from states of imbalance to states of equilibrium, insofar as it wants to conform to a primordial model; and it uses rites and rituals for this purpose. These rituals can be direct social ones, whose social utility results from the very practice of the ritual. Thus, for some, the prohibition of Muslims from eating pork would have had the direct social purpose of avoiding diseases contracted through the consumption of this meat. More precisely, the realization that there was a link between these diseases and pork gave rise to this Muslim ritual. One of the five pillars of Islam consists of the legal alms, the *zaka*. This is a contribution, in kind or in cash, which is paid by the Muslim to a mutual aid and charity fund, or even to cover certain public expenses. Some Muslim countries have retained this ritual, although only devout Muslims continue to consider themselves obliged to pay the *zaka*. This ritual of relief has played an important social role in the cohesion of Muslim communities, especially since these funds could only be used by Muslims. Today, the *zaka* is held up as an example by those who want to highlight the socialist character of Islam.

5.5.3. *Rituals of inversion*

Rituals of inversion are interesting because they have an indirect social influence. Thus, festivals are not only recreational, insofar as they momentarily free us from the need to repress impulses. The role of carnivals, for example, is to allow the human being to do what is forbidden. The rituals of celebration are above all rituals of inversion: inversion of social relations, derision of the powerful, contestation of power and questioning of the learned.

The behavior of people after the end of the lockdown period is essentially a ritual of inversion. These rituals of inversion can be analyzed along two axes, which are referred to in the literature as the "feast of the donkey" and the *Carmina Burana*. During the feast of the donkey, a bishop-buffoon was appointed and the subdeacons played cards and dice under the eyes of the officiating priest. This feast, in a way, was an organized reversal of the most sacred values. In 1444, the Faculty of Theology of Paris justified this festival by considering that the wine barrels would burst if the bunghole was not opened from time to time to air them. During the feast of the donkey, people indulged in antics for a few days so they could then devote themselves to the service of God with greater fervor. Is it not significant that this type of festival is currently resurfacing in various French regions (even if Covid-19 will force the cancellation of most of these festive gatherings), at a time when the Church is hardening its stance and noting a decline in religious practices?

The significance of the *Carmina Burana* is somewhat similar to that of the donkey festival. They were originally important literary texts in medieval Germany. The present-day listener of these works, especially in the work of composer Carl Orff, is caught and enchanted, and led into an obsessive and irresistible atmosphere. Fluctuating between rigor and magic, between fidelity to tradition and a revolt-like taste for innovation, the rituals of inversion ultimately have the effect of purifying the social system by overcoming the dissolving forces of society.

5.5.4. *Fighting the ritual with disorder*

The ritual festival also revives the youth of the world. There is a kind of mythical, timeless time that is embodied in the festival which can be an occasion to manifest the sacredness of the norms of everyday social life through their ritual violation. This is still the case today with the Rio carnival (Brazil) or, in France, the Dunkirk carnival (in the Nord department). The ritual festival is disorder, the overturning of prohibitions and social measures. It is a fusion in an immense fraternity, as opposed to the common social life that classifies and separates. In any case, order emerges regenerated from the festival, not only because we are tired of it, of its weight, but also because the social order wears itself out. In order to form what is rightly called a society, people feel the need to return to their origins in order to be reborn somewhere rejuvenated. However, it is true that here we are touching on an idealized conception of the ritual festival, especially since there are ritual festivals, not of protection, but of opposition.

5.5.5. *Rituals of opposition*

The use of rituals is sometimes used to limit or challenge the power and status quo of the order. The youth of May 1968 used certain rituals, including wearing their hair long and refusing to wear traditional clothing. These were rituals because ever since that time, young people who want to oppose and refuse society proceed in the same way, through rituals that can be called anti-conformist. Sporting rituals are also often those of opposition, which are all the more understandable in that they are linked to regional traditions, for example, Catalan traditions in the case of thirteen-a-side rugby in France. The demand in certain French regions, such as Brittany or Occitanie, to relearn the Breton or Occitan language in schools, is also a ritual of opposition because language can be considered a ritual. All of these reactions against a stifling order thus refused are themselves creators of order. While rituals usually mark the unity and identity of an ethnic-national community, oppositional rituals most often reflect a primarily ethnic-regional or communal unity and identity (e.g. hippie communities). Oppositional rituals are always, at the same time, destructive of an imposed social order and constructors of another social order that is felt and experienced. This is why the national order reacts against these types of rituals and why voices are raised to limit or even prohibit them.

5.5.6. *Integrated rituals*

The best way to block the desire for autonomy or the refusal of a social straitjacket expressed by rituals is to integrate them by means of national recognition. Politicians and diplomats very often resort to this in order to stop certain autonomist or rebellious impulses expressed through the resurgence of particularist rituals.

The corrida is the epitome of the attempted killing of an animal in public, in this case a bull. In France, the *Conseil d'Etat*, whose role is to advise the State on law-making, has recognized the legitimacy of certain regional ritual customs. It has thus considered that bullfights can be legally authorized in municipalities where they correspond to an uninterrupted local tradition. The legislator therefore intervened to modify the law of July 2, 1850, known as the Grammont law, in order to repress the ill-treatment of domestic animals. The law of November 19, 1963 maintained this offence and made it subject to correctional penalties but expressly excluded bullfights – and cockfights – from these penalties in regions where these ritual activities correspond to an uninterrupted local tradition. In this way, the central political power protects itself from reviving rituals that might be manifestations of opposition, while requiring that animal fighting rituals, in order to be legalized, not be interrupted at certain times. Transmuted into an ambiguous function, which retains enough oppositional power to keep these animal rituals attractive – and to prevent the desire for opposition from being transferred to other rituals – these rituals finally appear to be sufficiently integrated into the overall society, so that their disorganizing character is eliminated.

The second means of integrating rituals is punishment. Although Western societies today no longer have criminal sanctions for violating rituals, as was the case in China (where harmony between humanity and the general order of the world was advocated in all aspects of life), the social group as a whole nevertheless tends to reject those who do not intend to observe the rituals. This internalized rejection leads to a feeling of guilt on the part of the person who crosses the line; and through this sanction, which is not a sanction as such but which makes a mark on people's minds, the social order defends itself and succeeds in obtaining the respect, at least apparent, for the rituals it wishes to preserve.

5.6. Death and culture

In the field of death, culture is the bearer of many rituals. Corsican, Italian, Spanish and Portuguese women traditionally dress in black following the loss of a close relative, and they do so for the rest of their lives. This ritual is deeply rooted in Mediterranean culture. However, is there a systematic link between mortuary rituals and culture?

5.6.1. *Forms of interrogation*

It is possible to question the nature of the links between rituals and culture. It is not a question here of defining a notion as complex as culture, which we know to be very hazardous. Rather, we need to consider the relationship between the traditional and active elements of rituals and people's sense of their own culture in a given social system. In any case, cultures allow people to situate themselves, thus fulfilling one of the functions of rituals.

Rituals and festivals are all elements of culture and borrow certain characteristics from it. Certainly, in the case of religion, for example, there are many analogies in terms of rituals. They can be explained by the fact that human beings seem to have generic techniques of expression and symbols capable of expressing spontaneously, bypassing the conscious mind, this or that concept. This short-circuiting is even more important through digital tools. If we look at eating rituals, we can see that one-third of the planet eats with knives and forks, one-third with chopsticks and one-third with their hands, while all three of these populations use the same type of cell phone that has become a smartphone.

5.6.2. *Halloween: the manipulated birth of a ritual*

It has been pointed out above that certain rituals tend to disappear and that the sense of the sacred is lost, so perhaps the same should be true of the festivals and cultures associated with these rituals. For a certain period, which seems to be over, because of the resurgence of oppositional rituals, popular and regional cultures did decline. One of the consequences of the development of the mass media – and the separation of the elite from the rest of society – is that culture is now only a minority affair. In industrialized societies, culture is experienced as a kind of privilege and is used as an instrument of political struggle. Thus, the technological and computer advance in the United States has had the effect of destroying Western culture – with its rituals and traditions – and replacing it with American culture, particularly through data banks and "key events". The most visible phenomenon in this respect is the disappearance of the November weekend dedicated to the dead and the famous Day of the Dead on November 2, which have been replaced by the celebration of Halloween, through media and advertising images.

One question that arises is that of understanding whether the digitalization of societies can be the trigger for the creation of new rituals that will endure. To this end, it may be interesting to analyze the creation of Halloween. Initially, Halloween was a Celtic festival, of Gallic and Irish origin, whose tradition spread to the United States at the end of the 19th century. The Celtic year traditionally ended at the junction of October and November, and the last night of the year was the night of the God of Death (Samain or Samhain), the day on which the God of Death was supposed to inform the year's dead of their new destination or reincarnation. Halloween is, in fact, an American shortening of the expression *All Hallows Eve*, which literally means "the evening of all the saints", or the eve of All Saints' Day, which thus corresponds to October 31:

> According to Halloween's detractors, this commercial holiday of American origin has no business being celebrated in Europe without Anglo-Saxon ancestry. At best, it has been reduced to a derisory children's festival, during which kids go door to door begging for candy, and to a simple costume party with a macabre imagery of more than doubtful taste. At worst, Halloween is denounced as a despicable manifestation of Yankee cultural imperialism, and even as the expression of a disturbing upsurge of satanic subversion, whose hidden but obvious goal would be to annihilate and replace our traditional and Christian All Saints' Day[2].

However, the reality of the birth of Halloween is quite different and purely commercial. Philippe Cahen, a prospective consultant, imported the Anglo-Saxon festival to France by registering the Halloween trademark in

2 Retrieved and translated from: https://www.lengadoc-info.com/5736/histoire-et-tradition/halloween-fete-commerciale-identitaire.

1995 through his company Optos-Opus, following a trip to New York and the ideas that this trip gave him (Cahen 2000): a brand that commercialized confectionery, drinks, cakes and various food products. Following complaints from the unions of candy and cake manufacturers, the company lost its right to use the Halloween trademark after a now-famous ruling by the Commercial Chamber of the French Supreme Court in 2004. This ruling had significant indirect consequences, insofar as it is no longer possible to appropriate the names of villages and festivals in France as URLs for Internet sites. Today, Halloween is a more or less moribund phenomenon in France, whose interest remains fairly confidential, even if candy merchants still try to capitalize on the event. So, it seems very difficult to artificially create new rituals.

5.6.3. *Conjuring death*

The symbol allows the ritual to make sensible and acceptable what may not be, and it is a representation that must be understood not as it is immediately available to us, but through a wider meaning. Rituals usually have underlying symbols just as, conversely, some symbols are the source of rituals.

In order to ward off the signs of a possible new death, resurgence and new, "first time" festivals (Easter, Nowruz, Chinese New Year) are present in many societies, with the aim of staging a symbolically recreated new youth. Moreover, on an image placed on Facebook, it is possible to read the following comments: "Beautiful illustration of death"; "Superb… magnificent… nature amazes me. It dies and lives again. I'm in love with it"; "When the tree looks dead, everything is white"[3]. In fact, the symbolic ritual does not signify, but instead evokes and focuses on things other than "real death". Thus, this attitude assembles and concentrates a multiplicity of meanings, not reducing itself to a single, absolute and definitive meaning, but assembling itself to ward off death, without obstructing the feeling of fragility of our existences.

The feeling of existential fragility pushes people to lower themselves and to repress any movement of pride during the mortuary rituals. The Christian shows their deference by joining their hands during prayers. Deference does

3 Comments noted on Facebook in September and October 2019 in French.

not necessarily mean a relationship with a deity defined as superior to humans. Buddhists also join their hands, like Christians, as a sign of respect for another human being considered in an equal relationship. For them, this gesture does not symbolize a state of inferiority of human nature, but the basic principle of the ritual remains the notion of humility. The symbolic effectiveness of a ritual presupposes that everyone can recognize the symbol as such, that there is no dispute as to its abstract meaning. It is on this condition that the ritual has a value for the group, for the community, for society, that it has the power to gather people, to establish consensus. It preserves a certain freedom of acceptance of its meaning. It remains a flexible social value, in the sense that the symbolic ritual can be adapted to different social, economic and religious contexts, while retaining a spiritual dimension, an identical unconscious feeling.

5.7. Example of the handshake

The example of the handshake, which has now become forbidden in personal relationships following Covid-19, is very striking in this analysis of rituals. Indeed, there are a few social practices and few cultural behaviors that are not as imbued with symbolic rituals as the handshake. Fashion, advertising and architecture are all bearers of this symbolism. This is why it is possible to affirm that, conversely, every ritual is itself impregnated with the context in which it is performed. Thus, the handshake – with time and the evolution of the society in which it is performed – has taken on different meanings while remaining a ritual of agreement and encounter. From the first manifestation of the handshake, which corresponded to the fact that one presented oneself without weapons, it later signified that the meeting was not intended to be aggressive. Later, this ritual took on a positive meaning. Today, this gesture symbolizes a friendly encounter, a certain warmth, a certain pleasure. Even in special contexts, such as diplomatic meetings, the handshake ultimately symbolizes agreement.

Thus, after signing the armistice of June 22, 1940 in the forest of Compiègne (Oise), General Huntzinger for France and General Keitel for Germany shook hands to seal the agreement of their nations. In terms of this idea of agreement, the handshake in Montoire (Loir-et-Cher) between Marshal Pétain and Hitler, on October 24, 1940, is even more significant, because the principle of collaboration with Germany was admitted there. The symbolic ritual is an indirect means of communication, which only takes on its full value in a particular context, space and moment, insofar as it is necessarily intermediated by the social structure. The disappearance of the handshake ritual, as imposed by the social distancing advocated as a means of reducing the risk of contamination by the SARS-CoV-2 virus, perhaps puts into perspective the idea that we do not agree on what – and why – on each occasion.

5.8. Political rituals

The scepter or crown not only signals power but invites respect for it. Signs representing military ranks involve ritual attitudes such as saluting that symbolize hierarchical dependence. These ritual gestures prescribe reflexes of obedience and dependence. This is why, in a setting as closed and structured as the army, the role of injunction and prescription can be identified.

As a result of Covid-19, the political ritual is also reversed. It is the "people from below" who are put forward, and it is the "unworthy" who become the "leaders", the "front lines" and the respectable. Garbage collectors, nurses' aides, firefighters and cashiers become more than ever those on whom we depend, while not having to obey their orders, which is a remarkable nuance.

This conditioning through rituals is all the more sensitive as it is brutal and imposed. It is interesting to note that in the case of an imposition, the symbolic aspect of the rituals performed loses its importance. The more the symbolic aspect of a ritual plays a role, the more the attitude induced by the ritual joins the category of unconscious social and collective reflexes.

5.9. Conclusion

The tortuous journey, mysterious and anchored in daily life and societal functioning, which has just been accomplished through rituals, their subjects, their functions and their symbolic relations allows us to pose the following milestones, as elements of a conclusion to a questioning of the place of rituals in existence and its overcoming:

– the importance of rituals should not be underestimated, in terms of understanding the evolution of today's societies;

– ensuring a plurality of rituals is a guarantor of democracy in everyday life;

– it is advisable not to be too critical of rituals that appear outdated because these are reflections of a world that no longer exists;

– the ritual is a privileged instrument of culture, of perpetual questioning of the lay and the sacred, of humanity and society;

– the ritual guarantees a freedom of spirit if the conditions analyzed are met. This freedom, associated with a critical reflection on ourselves, inscribes humanity in history and allows progress in return.

5.10. References

Agamben, G. (2009). *"What is an Apparatus?" and Other Essays*. Stanford University Press, Palo Alto.

Akrich, M. (1998). Les utilisateurs, acteurs de l'innovation. *Éducation permanente*, 134.

Augé, M. (2008). *Où est passé l'avenir ?* Panama, Paris.

Bardini, T. (1996). Changement et réseaux sociotechniques, de l'inscription à l'affordance. *Réseaux*, 76, 127.

Bauman, Z. (2007). *S'acheter une vie*. Jacqueline Chambon Éditeur, Paris.

Bourdieu, P. (1979). *La Distinction, critique sociale du jugement*. Éditions de Minuit, Paris.

Bourdieu, P. (1982). *Ce que parler veut dire: L'économie des échanges linguistiques*. Fayard, Paris.

Bourdieu, P. (2003). *Méditation pascalienne*. Le Seuil, Paris.

Cahen, P. (1999). *Secrets et mystères d'Halloween*. Grancher, Paris.

Cahen, P. (2000). *Halloween le Guide. Des idées des recettes des déguisements*. LPM, Paris.

de Certeau, M. (1980). *L'invention du quotidien, Arts de faire*. UGE, Paris.

Chazal, G. (2006). *L'ordre humain: Ou le déni de nature*. Champ Vallon, Ceyzérieu.

El Hassani, J. (2021). Comment des personnes mortes peuvent-elles "liker" des choses sur Facebook ? *Slate* [Online]. Available at: http://www.slate.fr/lien/66037/personnes-mortes-like-facebook.

Ferraris, M. (2006). *T'es Où ? Ontologie du Téléphone mobile*. Albin Michel, Paris.

Fukuyama, F. (2012). *The End of History and the Last Man*. Penguin Books, London.

Gergen, K.J. (2002). The challenge of absent presence. In *Perpetual Contact*, Katz, J.E. and Aakhus, M. (eds). Cambridge University Press, Cambridge.

Giddens, A. (1994). L'émergence de la politique de vie. *Écologie Politique*, 11–12, 137–158.

Grossen, M. and Perret-Clermont, A.N. (1992). *L'espace thérapeutique. Cadres et contextes*. Delachaux, Neuchâtel and Niestlé, Paris.

Henderson, V. (1994). *La nature des soins infirmiers*. InterÉditions, Paris.

Huntington, S.P. (1993). The clash of civilizations? *Foreign Affairs, Council on Foreign Relations*, 72(3), 22–49.

Huntington, S.P. (2002). *The Clash Of Civilizations and the Remaking of World Order*. Simon & Schuster, London.

Ireland, C. (2009). Samuel Huntington, 81, political scientist, scholar. *The Harvard Gazette* [Online]. Available at: news.harvard.edu/gazette/story/2009/02/samuel-huntington-81-political-scientist-scholar/.

D'Iribarne, P. (1989). *La logique de l'honneur*. Le Seuil, Paris.

D'Iribarne, P. (2008). *Penser la diversité du monde*. Le Seuil, Paris.

Jacquard, A. (2005). *Nouvelle petite philosophie*. Stock, Paris.

Jouët, J. (2000). Retour critique sur la sociologie des usages. *Réseaux*, 18(100), 487–521.

Lévi-Straus, C. (1962). *La Pensée sauvage*. Plon, Paris.

Matellart, A. (2008). *La Globalisation de la surveillance – Aux origines de l'ordre sécuritaire*. La Découverte, Paris.

Morin, E. (2002). Au-delà de la globalisation et du développement, société monde ou empire monde ? Quelle autre mondialisation ? *Revue du Mauss*, 20, 43–53.

Ouest-France (2020). 1 000 noms de personnes décédées du Covid-19: La Une choc du New York Times. *Ouest-France* [Online]. Available at: https://www.ouest-france.fr/monde/etats-unis/1-000-noms-de-personnes-decedees-du-covid-19-la-une-choc-du-new-york-times-6844380.

Rifkin, J. (2000). *L'âge de l'accès, la nouvelle culture du capitalisme*. La Découverte, Paris.

Roqueplo, P. (1997). *Entre savoir et décision, l'expertise scientifique*. INRA, Paris.

Sardais, S. (2005). Leadership et création des institutions. Les actions, intentions et perceptions. PhD Thesis, HEC, Paris.

Stiegler, B. (2008). *Prendre soin, de la jeunesse et des générations*. Flammarion, Paris.

Venkatesh, V. (2000). Determinants of perceived ease of use: Integrating control, intrinsic motivation, and emotion into the technology acceptance model. *Information Systems Research*, 11(4), 342–365.

Vergely, B. (2003). *Petite philosophie pour jours tristes*. Milan éditions, Toulouse.

Veyne, P. (1971). *Comment on écrit l'histoire*. Le Seuil, Paris.

Virilio, P. (1984). *L'horizon négatif*. Galilée, Paris.

Voge, J. (1985). Crise, information et communication, avenir relatif des réseaux mailés et pyramidaux. *Communication & Medicin*e, 11(3), 61–72.

Voge, J. (1997). *Le complexe de Babel, crise ou maîtrise de l'information ?* Masson, Paris.

Winner, L. (1980). Do artefacts have politics? *Daedalus*, 109.

Wolton, D. (2003). *L'autre mondialisation*. Flammarion, Paris.

Zarifian, P. (2004). *L'échelle du monde. Globalisation, altermondialisme, mondialité*. La Dispute, Paris.

6

The New Innovators in the Footsteps of the Coronavirus

6.1. Introduction

Crises, chaos and changes have generated innovations throughout the ages and the history of humanity. New ways of thinking are constructed and, in these times of urgency, action takes precedence over reflection. The patterns of the past can no longer be applied, and it becomes essential to regenerate the individual and collective creative spirit (Weisberg 1993; Sternberg 2005). In this chapter, we propose to explore this regeneration of minds through the light of past experiences and with regard to the many innovative examples that are already emerging.

6.2. Pre-Covid innovators

Innovation is currently seen as positive and indispensable in companies, where all employees are now expected to be innovators. In 1750, innovation was not viewed positively when the *Encyclopédie ou Dictionnaire raisonné des sciences, des arts et des métiers,* edited by Diderot and d'Alembert, was published: the definition of innovation was as follows: "A new or important change made in the political government of a State against the usage and rules of its constitution. These kinds of innovation are always deformities in the political order."

Chapter written by Henri SAMIER, Emmanuel CHÉNÉ and Guy CAVEROT.

6.2.1. *Generations of innovation*

6.2.1.1. *Imitation*

In previous centuries, the quality of reproduction made the reputations of painters. As with art during the Renaissance (from the 14th to the 16th century and up to the mid-17th century), reproduction and imitation were valued activities, with the reproduction of scenes in paintings, including Leonardo da Vinci's Mona Lisa, being a good example.

A redirection took place with Art Nouveau (end of the 19th and beginning of the 20th century), with the focus less on reality than on the esthetics of lines and forms. Then came the expressionist and cubist painters in the first half of the 20th century, with Picasso, Braque and after that abstract art, then the surrealists, and finally the modernists. Then, artists appropriated photography in the 19th century and also diverted it, and finally cinema appeared, which also went through phases of imitation and then interpretation/distortion.

Today, copying is an activity decried in favor of innovation, which moves away from the subject to reinterpret, invent and disrupt and is increasingly valued.

6.2.1.2. *Technology combinations and transfers*

Combinations and cross-fertilization are often sources of innovation. The crossroads of technologies, as well as the crossroads of professions, are conducive to serendipity (the conjunction of chance). In this sense, history teaches us about the first gimmick in the history of cinema, the work of Georges Méliès, who introduced special effects completely by chance. After a problem during a projection, when the mechanism jammed, he started to turn the crank again and said that he then saw the men transformed into women and the bus transformed into a hearse! Whereas on the last recorded image, there was a bus, when Méliès resumed his projection, in the same place, there was a hearse. Illusion, the ancestor of special effects, was born. It is perhaps no coincidence that Georges Méliès, born in Paris in 1861, was an illusionist before becoming a film-maker, a profile of an innovator!

However, in business, innovators cannot wait for chance. They must provoke situations of serendipity (Prax 1997, pp. 157–158). To do this, they increasingly appropriate field research methods and come into contact with users, as well as other innovation disciplines: sociologies, semiologies, psychologies, etc. In this sense, open innovation encourages companies to work together with their counterparts or to find partners in order to develop technological innovations in a techno-push logic. Other transfers can be made in disjointed fields, such as Tao and physics (Capra 1975) or acoustics and biology (Henry 2015).

6.2.1.3. *Dissemination on the markets*

Innovators were also led to work outside the walls, following the example of the Impressionist painters (Renoir, Cézanne, etc.), with the innovation of the "gray tubes" that allowed painters to leave their studios, whether these walls were real or virtual. The development of photography at the same time also called into question the faithful representation of reality. Thus, in a market pull logic, the current approaches of design thinking and, more generally, use-based approaches allow practices to be brought to the fore. Previously, designers worked in research departments and interactions were rare. Innovators are increasingly gathering talent, and the approaches are also fed by the demands of the market. Science must finally integrate value-adding into its process, which is an important paradigm shift.

6.3. Types of innovators

6.3.1. *The explorer*

The innovator is basically an explorer, a discoverer like Christopher Columbus. Like the discovery of a continent, the invention is still raw; the innovator is in this sense an evangelist who will transform the raw material into a diamond. In this sense, innovation is often defined as an invention that has found its market. Jean-Yves Naouri[1] indicates that:

> For example, Sony was the inventor of the Walkman, and Kodak offered the best cameras. These brands, which were at the top, were caught up, overtaken and had to come back in other sectors. Kodak certainly invented digital photography in its laboratories in the 1970s, but it was too early. You have to

1 Chief Operating Officer of Publicis (2017). Les Matins de l'économie. *JDD*, June 20.

> keep ideas in your boxes and pull them out at the right time (Valiant 2017).

He goes on to say, regarding the innovator, that "you have to be at the intersection of IQ (intelligence quotient), TQ (technology quotient) and EQ (emotional quotient)". In a world where everything is accelerating, it is becoming important to work less on the result than on the process, and particularly on time, in order to reduce duration. The development of agile methods, design thinking and lean startup promote the notions of the draft, the "rough draft", iteration, etc., in order to gather user feedback upstream.

Moreover, gaining speed means allowing intuition to express itself. "Intuition is intelligence that is speeding", said French playwright Henry Bernstein (Landis 2009). On the other hand, it is not the same circuits of reflection that are mobilized; the mental ones will work in an analytical way, while the instinctive ones will work in a more intuitive way. As Henri Poincaré, a French mathematician, reminds us, "it is through logic that we prove, it is through intuition that we invent" (Morisson 2013).

6.3.2. *The rebel (disobedience and disorder)*

Innovators have to act disobedient in essence: disobedience with codes and rules… while remaining within a "cone of acceptability". According to Laurent Dassault, Chief Operating Officer of the Dassault Group:

> You always have to be one step ahead of your competitors, otherwise you die. So to innovate, you have to know how to take risks, but smart risks (Valiant 2017).

This is also reflected in management methods, so the innovator must disturb the established order and push back the limits of the system in which they evolve. This directly challenges the ability to manage an innovator in an organization. In the various management methods[2], the participatory approach is preferable for encouraging commitment and initiative and making management accountable and involving it in decision-making at a very early stage. This approach is essentially based on a culture that advocates delegation of power, communication and mutual respect. Indeed, all decisions are the result of a consensus between the various stakeholders.

2 Management that is directive, persuasive, participative and delegative.

6.3.3. *Corporate hacking*

Corporate hacking is the act of acting outside the rules of the company, more like a "rebel" and less like a "good soldier". It is difficult to give a definition to this trend which, if we were to explain it, would express "fixing", "tinkering", terms which are not very positive, whereas the approach is deeply positive. The innovative thing about it is that it can integrate generations Y and Z, who are the ones entering the organizations and who will quickly become the pillars of them (see the adventure of the hacktivators):

> Improvisation, positive diversion, and organizational tinkering: for the corporate hacker, almost any means are good for working, in the collective, to improve the company (Lomig 2016).

The idea of "bricolage" is emerging, with the Makers movement established and residing in several cities in France, concomitantly with the emergence of the concept of the quick-and-dirty, that is, a strategy or protocol elaborated with little care but having the advantage of being a quick way to solve a particular problem.

This trend is quite recent and is part of new methodologies such as frugal innovation, the circular economy and lean startups.

The importance of sketches, which were relevant for paintings during the Renaissance, is resurfacing in the sense of intermediate design objects. Even if imperfect, the product or service has the merit of existing. Teams gather valuable feedback, observe usage and can react quickly. These intermediate representations can be virtual at first and become increasingly tangible. They have two inseparable functions: to model reality in terms of the advanced notion of virtual reality and to enable coordination and cooperation between the project actors (Bassereau 1996).

6.4. In-Covid innovators (2020–2021)

6.4.1. *The birth of innovations in times of crisis*

The lockdown period was conducive, on the one hand, to the natural emergence of fears (Kessler 2004; André 2005; Chodron 2005) and, on the other hand, to the emergence of a collective and of group thinking (Esser 1998). In a face-to-face setting, a collaborator may be self-effacing, not daring to intervene. On the other hand, in a remote setting, they can express themselves without fear and take their place as equals, especially with more charismatic collaborators. In the remote mode, exchanges take place via platforms, which are particularly effective in structuring organized and capitalizable thought. Indeed, the tools used for collective actions (Adobe Connect, Discord, FramaPad, Google Docs, etc.) make it easier to distribute the word, as well as to keep track of the organized exchanges. All this contributes to a psycho-sociological phenomenon of consensus resulting from a group that meets to think and make a decision. The group thus gives itself the illusion of thinking collectively about a problem and reaching a common position resulting from individual and singular approaches, without them being paralyzed by poor group dynamics.

6.4.2. *Examples of innovations arising in times of crisis*

The concept of the quick-and-dirty was highlighted during the crisis, as early as January 2020, by various countries such as China and South Korea. As part of this approach in France, the work of Didier Raoult, for example, has been strongly criticized by the scientific community, with regard to the use of hydroxychloroquine coupled with azithromycin in the treatment of patients with Covid-19. The disagreements were about the efficacy of the antimalarial against the coronavirus: the opposition between two models. One advocates the testing a priori of a treatment that has been proven in other related contexts, and the other maintains that all scientific protocols must be followed. The former indicates to the latter that the validation of a treatment would only be possible when it is no longer needed! However, emergency or war situations require emergency measures and war innovations.

The Makers movement has also produced significant results during the crisis. There was the case of the breathing apparatus developed in a few weeks by a group of discoverers, pioneers and trailblazers who passed, in a transversal way, over hierarchies and organizations, promoting action to the detriment of protocol.

The Makers for Life collective was created ex nihilo in Nantes to develop an artificial respirator in record time. The MakAir respirator[3] is an inexpensive, collaborative, open source project that can be produced on a large scale. It was the first university project supported by the French

3 For more information, please visit https://makair.life.

Ministry of the Armed Forces, following a call for projects on March 19, 2020 concerning innovative solutions to combat the Covid-19 pandemic. More than 2,500 proposals were received in this context. The MakAir respirator project particularly caught the attention of the French Defense Innovation Agency (*Agence d'innovation de défense*, AID), said the University of Nantes[4]. The project was supported by the University of Nantes through its subsidiary *Capacités* and by the Nantes University Hospital with the Makers For Life collective[5]. Starting with 5 people, 150 were mobilized after 10 days. Backed by the University Hospital, the university and the French Alternative Energies and Atomic Energy Commission (*Commissariat à l'énergie atomique et aux énergies alternatives*, CEA), the project was supported by local authorities and international industrialists.

In addition to the researchers, the team was organized around a group of business leaders, students and employees of small- and medium-sized enterprises, as well as large groups and also public–private crossovers in the association of two regions: Pays de la Loire and Auvergne-Rhône-Alpes. Overall, more than 250 people were involved in the project:

> In five weeks, an alliance of academics and doctors supported by an ecosystem of start-ups designed an open source respirator with the help of the Atomic Energy Commission[6].

In this context, action took precedence over reflection. The university, known for training Cartesian minds, was a stakeholder and even the support of the project, a paradox a priori since the Makers movement calls on people who are involved in action, breaking with "pure" university training, which is protocol-structured around Cartesian minds. However, this is not the only paradox.

An unprecedented human, technological and scientific adventure was created in a race against time to finalize, in five weeks, a respirator that could be industrialized. The 3D plans allowed the prototypes to be made with 3D printing and assembly of commercially available components. Parts

---

4 See the article on the university's website at: https://fondation.univ-nantes.fr/accueil/covid-19-fabrication-de-respirateurs-artificiels-reglementaires-2620481.kjsp.

5 For more information on this subject, please visit https://vipress.net/le-collectif-francais-makers-for-life-prepare-la-production-du-respirateur-makair/.

6 See https://www.lemonde.fr/campus/article/2020/04/20/entre-nantes-et-grenoble-une-course-contre-la-montre-pour-creer-un-respirateur-artificiel-a-bas-cout_6037140_4401467.html.

were thus produced thanks to the mobilization of numerous 3D printers in laboratories, as well as in several companies in the Nantes region. After validation, the idea was to make the plans available to all, as open source. In this way, these respirators could be manufactured all over the world. The company SEB offered to manufacture them industrially, along with other large companies that joined the project, such as Renault, Michelin, HP and STMicroelectronics[7].

6.4.3. *Motivations of innovators*

Innovators may have motivations that stem from their personal histories, their upbringings or their deepest aspirations. We can draw a parallel between innovators and geniuses, who are outstanding innovators who mark their times. Throughout history, the nine identified characteristics of genius[8] (Aristotle, Mozart, Einstein, Picasso, Elon Musk, etc.) are presented in Box 6.1.

1) Original, open-minded, free of convention and able to put into perspective and deconstruct problems.

2) Aware of what is going on, what changes are occurring and what patterns are emerging.

3) Analytical, able to solve problems logically.

4) Creative, open to possibilities and using the "what if" game to solve problems.

5) Synergistic, inclined to think in parallel, tolerating ambiguities and connecting new links.

6) Prolific, able to generate many creative ideas or solutions.

7) Pragmatic, aware of the need to transform theories and concepts into practices and realities.

8) Visionary, able to communicate holistically, symbolically and without words.

9) Personal trust, which can be found in the human element (Schutz 2006).

Box 6.1. *Characteristics of innovators*

7 See https://www.lesechos.fr/industrie-services/automobile/respirateurs-artificiels-ce-que-font-vraiment-les-constructeurs-automobiles-1190557.

8 "Are you the Einstein or Picasso of business?" by Peter Fisk, at: https://www.thegeniusworks.com/wp-content/uploads/2017/04/Einstein-and-Picasso-by-Peter-Fisk.pdf.

All innovators have these nine characteristics to a greater or lesser extent, while geniuses have them strongly developed. It is all a question of intensity. An author specializing in the mind map (Buzan 1994) adds the "genius quotient", which he defines as the intelligence of singularity, very valuable in times of crisis.

In parallel, a model of the "seven I's" has been developed (Samier 2018), which defines the characteristics (skills, abilities and aptitudes) of innovators as: inspiration, imagination (Laborit 1993), intelligence, insouciance, intuition (Choquette 2018), illusion and invisibility. In this pandemic period, insouciance and illusion are perhaps less present in favor of the other five. Moreover, intelligence was solicited, when rather it should have been intelligences that were solicited in the sense of the 12 forms of intelligence, namely: logical, linguistic, musical, spatial, kinesthetic, intrapersonal, existential, interpersonal, spiritual, naturalistic, singular and intuitive.

Certain intelligences are "harmed" or less stimulated during periods of forced isolation, such as kinesthetic intelligence (contact and touch) and interpersonal intelligence (the relationship with others in a face-to-face setting), which also includes emotional intelligence (Goleman 1995).

Naturally, in times of crisis, it is essential to develop our relationship with ourselves and to practice meditation (Loizzo 2014) in order to tame our stress (Fradin 2010) and to calm the thinker (Marquis 2005), that is, the mind that can run in a loop.

6.4.3.1. *Urgency and the need to react: the reason for urgency*

In the Covid-19 crisis, ways of thinking, communicating and acting are constrained by time, and saving time means saving lives.

The urgency to react locally in a global context shows us the difficulties of communication in the hyperconnected world where everyone has an opinion and everyone knows in part that everyone knows or is informed of what is happening on the planet.

The catalytic effect of the crisis is visible in the health sector where professionals are all united in sharing experiences and good practices in order to reduce the number of victims and shorten the duration of the pandemic.

In the midst of the emergency, people of goodwill spontaneously emerge to contribute and make a difference. This can be seen on many levels: from volunteers providing assistance, to the makers of visors and masks, to bloggers who spread the word on their channels. There are many examples of the creativity, responsiveness and inventiveness of individuals, groups and companies.

For example, Aviointeriors, an Italian aeronautical design company, has come up with aircraft design solutions[9] that respect social distancing and ensure the protection and safety of travelers for post-pandemic air travel.

Hackaton Covid, a programming marathon, has brought forth streamlined operational solutions, such as:

– *Innomed360.com*: a secure website that calculates in real time the number of beds available in health-care institutions.

– *Quick-help.app*: a website that connects volunteers who want to help people with shopping, babysitting, going to the pharmacy, etc.

Other sites identify significant innovations related to the Covid-19 crisis[10] (Figure 6.1).

Finally, the European Commission jointly organized hackathons, such as the EUvsVirus Hackathon[11]. In the first stage, the jury identified 117 solutions out of 2,160 ideas to fight the coronavirus epidemic. One example is Team Discover, which concerns a pair of glasses that measure a patient's temperature, oxygen saturation and breathing[12]. In a second step, all winners competed in a Matchathon, which took place from May 22 to 25, 2020 on the new EIC Covid[13] platform.

---

9 For more information, read the article at: https://www.departures.com/travel/aviointeriors-debuts-new-shielded-airplane-seat-designs.

10 See, for example, https://www.covidinnovations.com/.

11 For more information, please visit https://euvsvirus.org/results/.

12 For more information, please visit https://devpost.com/software/team-discover-qg7kn3.

13 For more information, please see https://ec.europa.eu/info/funding-tenders/opportunities/portal/screen/covid-19.

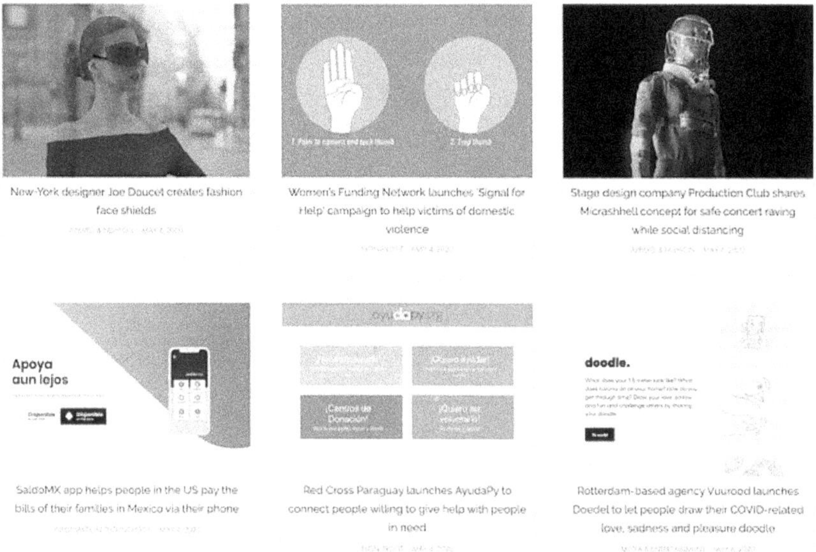

Figure 6.1. *More than 600 "Covid innovations" identified (source: www.covidinnovations.com)*

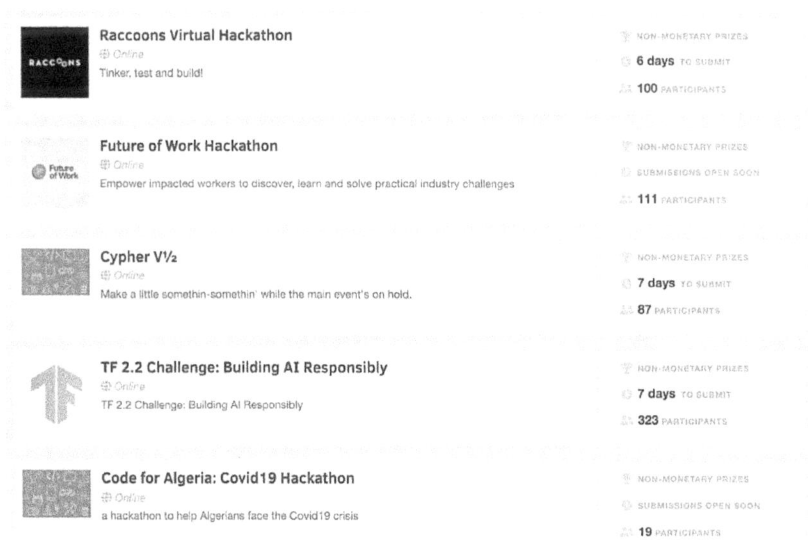

Figure 6.2. *Current hackathons (source: devpost.com)*

The emergency has also led to the emergence of innovation challenges and competitions such as:

– *COVID-19 Detect and Protect Challenge*: the United Nations Development Programme[14] (UNDP) and Hackster.io, an online open source technology community, have launched an innovation challenge to detect and protect against Covid-19. The idea is to create an open source technology that developing countries can use in the fight against this pandemic.

– *Hack the Crisis*[15]: this is a virtual collaboration of talents aiming to go from idea to useful prototype in 48 hours.

In an emergency, responses are short-term and time-constrained. Long-term visions and reflections will follow after these operational actions. We can also mention four more hackathon challenges: those of the HEC, the École Polytechnique and Science Po[16] and the Swiss Versus Virus[17] Hackathon.

6.4.3.2. *Duty, gift or sacrifice*

During lockdown, we (the authors of this text) decided individually and as innovators to experience a week of sacrifice by fasting. The three of us, each in our own way, prepared ourselves mentally, physically and spiritually for this fast. This symbolic experience of austerity, introspection and rest for the body brought us to a standstill. At least, our digestive systems came to a standstill, as if to signify that in the future we would not swallow any physical, emotional and spiritual food.

In this experiment, experienced by each of us, we were able to see the regenerating benefits of fasting in terms of the body, spirit and our relationship with others[18]. This time also allowed us to learn about the benefits of fasting[19].

14 For more information, please visit https://www.undp.org/content/undp/en/home/news-centre/news/2020/undp-and-hackster-io-partner-to-launch-a-global-innovation-chall.html.

15 For more information, see https://www.agorize.com/fr/challenges/hackthecrisisfrance?lang=en.

16 For more information, please visit https://hackingcovid19.fr/challenges/.

17 For more information, please visit https://www.versusvirus.ch.

18 For more information, see https://www.chuv.ch/fileadmin/sites/glg/documents/glg_symposium_gastro-enterologymici_feb2016_mottet.pdf.

19 For more information, see https://www.inserm.fr/sites/default/files/2017-11/Inserm_ThematicReport_YouthEffectiveness_2014.pdf.

6.4.3.3. *Pivoting*

In the energy sector, the Danish company Orsted (formerly Dong Energy) made a change more than 10 years ago from oil to wind energy. Today, this group is the leader in offshore wind energy and has the ambition to operate solely on green energy in order to eventually decarbonize Denmark and, why not, Europe. This exemplary demonstration of accessible technologies paves the way to new fields of research and innovation and helps to meet the great challenge of post-Covid-19 energy.

6.4.3.4. *New mindset: change to the unknown*

Let us take the example of the co-founder of the DoYouBuzz.com website, Ludovic Simon, who embodies a new spirit of inventiveness or a new psychology of innovation (Dukan 2006). Six months ago, Ludovic Simon moved with his family from Nantes to Saillans, a small village in the Drôme region. A total change of ecosystem, a leap into the unknown, and on April 30, 2020, he resigned as president of DoYouBuzz during the lockdown period and sold his shares in the company to the team that was running it. He said his final goodbye six months after jumping ship and wrote a goodbye message to his former colleagues[20]:

> In a few words, today we live differently, more soberly, with a much stronger link with nature. Time passes more slowly, we eat better and take care of our bodies, we have a different relationship with others too, perhaps more serene and deeper. In short, I feel that I belong here, in Saillans. This valley is a fabulous field of experimentation to LIVE today and to prepare tomorrow in the best possible conditions. A new chapter in my life has just opened up.

6.5. Post-Covid innovators

6.5.1. *Sense and common sense*

Covid-19, by placing people in a context of isolation, has led them to reflect and also demonstrated, in broad daylight, the activities that are essential to humanity: producing, transforming and distributing in order to

20 The full letter (in French) is available at: https://medium.com/@ludosim/goodbye-goodbye-pr%C3%A9sident-f4a5dd8844e1.

feed; protecting and caring in order to save; reflecting in order to act. Sensitivity to the "meaning of things", as Jacques Attali calls it (Attali 2009), is back. A few years before Covid-19, a search for meaning in economic activities was already emerging because of, among other things, the lack of understanding of employees about their work, the incoherence between life on the ground and governance and the loss of "common" sense in the decisions taken. Thus, meaning is regained and the future is looked at with a view to a better world.

In this context, innovators are following a common sense logic, in which useful innovations meet real social and societal needs. The speed of the crisis therefore raised the question of meaning (meaning and direction). It is mentally and deeply that we are questioned about:

– Why am I doing this?

– How do I want to change things?

–With whom do I want to co-create?

Every innovator must answer these three questions about meaning, direction or chosen trajectory and the collective.

6.5.2. *Collective and remote working tools*

For the past 30 years, major innovations have been developed in a collaborative manner between end-users (large companies, public services), technology suppliers (SMEs), knowledge producers (laboratories, private research centers) and other players facilitating the emergence of innovation (competitiveness clusters, regions). This trend, which is already well established, for example, in the European research framework (H2020, Horizon Europe) and the French framework (PSPC, ANR), will develop further. From now on, innovation will benefit from the massive use of collaborative work tools that have proven their worth during lockdown (Microsoft Teams, Zoom Meetings, BigBlueButton, Effi'connect). These tools enable effective remote working and will bring about new sustainable practices (Scharmer 2013). They will make it possible to enlist more remote partners and will undoubtedly optimize the methodologies for the emergence of the collective work necessary for innovative creation.

6.5.3. *Balance of activity–nature–assessment*

Innovations are characterized by their impacts in terms of value creation such as economic activity (turnover, gross domestic product, profits), the production of intellectual property (patents, models), the emergence of strategic positions (creation of sectors) and the social improvement brought about by innovations. Until now, the expected impacts were focused on the economic and strategic dimensions. The strong awareness of the need to take into account our environment and the key activities of our society during lockdown will undoubtedly lead to the redirection of these impacts towards human well-being, respect for the environment and social balance. This choice of a new direction for innovations will lead to the consideration, from the design of projects, of the response to tangible needs and the embedding of the products of innovations in a natural and social environment. These impacts will also have to be consistent with industrial, economic and social public policies.

6.5.4. *Innovations for humans*

Future innovations will tend to serve basic human needs. Thus, the fields of innovation will be oriented towards better nutrition to produce better quality food. For example, in agronomy, robotics will develop to replace chemical weed killers and thus, myriads of robots will be used to mechanically weed fields, and, other robot-drones will identify weeds, in order to target the necessary chemical weeding. The lack of manpower for fruit picking will probably also lead to the use of new machines. For strawberry and tomato picking, for example, automated systems will make it possible to harvest in compliance with health regulations without touching the fruit and vegetables with human hands. The processing of products will also be modified in order to produce food that is healthier or has a lower negative impact on nature.

6.5.5. *Organizational innovations*

Undeniably, lockdown showed the possibility of generalizing remote work. Until now, this mode of working was limited in companies, but lockdown has shown that it is possible to maintain efficiency in work while employing telematic means. The use of remote working on a larger scale will allow companies to make significant gains in office space and will also allow employees to work even if they live far away from the company. New forms of contract will undoubtedly emerge, offering activities almost exclusively carried out remotely. In addition, European regions that have been neglected because they are far from large cities or major traffic routes will probably develop and introduce remote working units, bringing together employees from different companies. This new distribution of workers, or rather, of the workforce, will be the result of a number of changes in the way in which they are distributed. This new distribution of workers, or rather remote workers, over the territory will have the consequence of reducing the ecological impact linked to car travel.

6.5.6. *Technical innovations*

Technical innovations will remain, but they will be developed in a different way in order to fit into economic schemes that are less oriented towards short-term performance and the over-consumption of fossil resources. We can imagine that frugal innovation, which has been quite rare until now, will be more present thanks to Covid-19. For example, in industry, the refurbishment of machines will be favored, rather than the systematic replacement of the means of production. Innovations will be created based on the renovation of functional elements that are still operational. By integrating new technologies, the operation of machines can be improved. This will also be a strong trend for the usual consumer goods of Europeans. For example, in the future, we can imagine making modifications to our car when the bodywork is still functional, by integrating electric engines and replacing the driving interfaces with more efficient modules (GPS, driving assistance systems, etc.).

6.6. Conclusion

New innovators will hybridize existing models and create new agile and sustainable methods with reference to the future. Going all digital will not be enough, neither will going all local. The blue economy (Pauli 2019) is, in this respect, a very inspiring idea. It is indeed an innovative economy that encourages the use of what is locally available and its distribution, both digitally and in a reasoned way, and one that does not produce side effects for the planetary ecosystem. This idea will be the new norm, although it will take time to get the international community on board. Many authors have foreseen the end of a civilization model and the emergence of a new world.

Among them are Marc Luyckx Ghisi[21], with a new civilization (Luyckx Ghisi 2010; Goux-Baudiment 2018); Marc Halevy, with a paradigm shift that comes with a trigger (the butterfly effect) and a so-called "snowball" amplifier (Halevy 2019); and Michel Bauwens (Bauwens 2015) and his peer-to-peer model, which is proving to be robust in the context of the health crisis. Finally, even if the five prospective scenarios (Futurible 2020) are not very optimistic, we share the firm belief and hope that the new post-Covid innovators will be fervent optimists[22], bold and humanistic.

6.7. References

André, C. (2005). *Psychologie de la peur: Craintes, angoisses et phobies*. Poche, Paris.

Attali, J. (2009). *Le sens des choses*. Robert Laffont, Paris.

Bassereau, J.-F., Charvet Pello, R., Faucheu, J., Delafosse, D. (1996). Les objets intermédiaires de conception / design, instruments d'une recherche par le design. *Sciences du Design*.

Bauwens, M. (2015). *Sauver le monde: Vers une économie post-capitalisme avec le peer-to-peer*. Les liens qui libèrent, Paris.

Buzan, T. and Keene, R. (1994). *Buzan's Book of Genius and How to Unleash Your Own*. Stanley Paul and Co Ltd, London.

Capra, F. (1975). *The Tao of Physics*. Shambhala Publications, Boulder.

Chodron, P. (2005). *Les bastions de la peur*. Pocket, Paris.

Choquette, S. (2018). *Vos trois supers pouvoirs: Méditation, imagination et intuition*. Exergues, Paris.

Dukan, L. (2006). Psychology of innovation and change factors. In *Innovation Engineering: The Power of Intangible Networks*, Corsi, P., Christofol, H., Richir, S., Samier, H. (eds). ISTE Ltd, London and Wiley, New York.

Fradin, J. (2010). *L'intelligence du stress*. Eyrolles, Paris.

Futurible (2020). Crise du Covid-19: Scénarios à l'horizon fin 2020 [Online]. Available at: https://www.futuribles.com/fr/document/crise-du-covid-19-esquisse-de-scenarios-a-lhorizon/.

21 Thinkerview (2017). Changement de Civilisation ? Marc Luyckx Ghisi [EN DIRECT] [Online]. Available at: https://www.youtube.com/watch?v=JDRzEdRQF5s.

22 *Ligue des optimistes website*, see: https://www.liguedesoptimistes.fr.

Goleman, D. (1995). *Emotional Intelligence*. Bantam, New York.

Goux-Baudiment, F. (2018). *La Grande Transition de l'humanité: De Sapiens à Deus*. FYP éditions, Limoges.

Gunther Pauli, G. (2019). *L'Économie bleue 3.0*. Édition de l'Observatoire, Paris.

Halevy, M. (2019). *Maîtriser le changement: La révolution économique*, Volume 1. Transitions Éditions, London.

Henry, M. (2015). *De l'information à l'exformation*. Association Natur'Eau Quant, Saint-Cézaire-sur-Siagne.

Kesser, J. (1998). Alive and well after 25 years: A review of groupthink research. *Organizational Behavior and Human Decision Processes*, 73(2–3), 116–141.

Kessler, D. and Kubler-Ross, E. (2004). *Leçons de vie: Comprendre le sens de nos désirs, de nos peurs et de nos espoirs*. Pocket, Paris.

Laborit, H. (1993). *L'homme imaginant*. 10/18, Paris.

Landis, J. (2009). *Le Théâtre d'Henry Bernstein*. L'Harmattan, Paris.

Loizzo, J. (2014). Meditation research, past, present, and future: Perspectives from the Nalanda contemplative science tradition. *Advances in Meditation Research: Neuroscience and Clinical Applications*, 1307, 43–54.

Lomig (2016). Corporate Hacking: Qu'est-ce que c'est ? *Les hacktivateurs* [Online]. Available at: https://hacktivateurs.co/2016/04/05/corporate-hacking-quest-ce-que-cest/.

Luyckx Ghisi, M. (2010). *Surgissement d'un nouveau monde: Valeurs, vision, économie*. Alphée, Monaco.

Marquis, S. (2015). *On est foutu, on pense trop! Comment se libérer de Pensouillard le hamster*. Éditions de la Martinière, Paris.

Morisson, J. (2013). *Intuition et 6e sens: Une enquête aux frontière de la psychologie*. Éditions de la Martinière, Paris.

Prax, J.Y. (1997). *Le taux de découverte et la sérendipité*. Insep Éditions, Paris.

Samier, H. (2018). *Intuition, Creativity, Innovation*. ISTE Ltd, London, and Wiley, New York.

Scharmer, O. and Kaufer, K. (2013). *Leading from the Emerging Future*. Berret-Koehler, San Francisco.

Schutz, W. (2006). *L'élément humain: Comprendre le lien entre estime de soi, confiance et performance*. InterEditions, Paris.

Sternberg, R.J. (2005). Creativity or creativities? *International Journal of Human–Computer Studies*, 63, 370–382.

Vaillant, G. (2017). L'innovation, c'est une invention qui a réussi [Online]. Available at: https://www.lejdd.fr/Economie/Les-Matins-de-l-economie-du-JDD-L-innovation-c-est-une-invention-qui-a-reussi-659132.

Weisberg, R.W. (1993). *Creativity: Beyond the Myth of Genius*. Freeman, New York.

7

Behavior and Anticipation of the Covid-19 Crisis

7.1. Preamble

The fact that the Covid-19 epidemic is still ongoing – and evolving in different ways in many different countries – means that there is still very little scientific synthesis work based on sufficient hindsight and objectivity that could be used to judge the behaviors that would have been necessary for curative anticipation of the Covid-19 crisis, i.e. anticipation that could permanently deal with Covid-19.

In the absence of detailed answers regarding the societal behaviors that could have been able to anticipate the pandemic produced by the SARS-CoV-2 virus, our discussion will therefore essentially consist of questions.

7.2. Anticipation, uncertainty and acceptability

Today, all public and private organizations are faced with increasingly frequent and complex crisis situations involving a growing number of people, both legal and physical. The health, societal, economic and geopolitical implications of these crisis situations, which are already considerable today, may become even more significant in the near future.

Chapter written by Christian SCHOEN.

In spite of the uncertainties and the risks of bad decisions that it implies, anticipation, which is in a way a societal obligation, implies adapted and coordinated organizational solutions with regard to the Covid-19 crisis and future close threats, all the more so as the triggering of a second epidemic wave seems possible, and this before the availability of a vaccine (or better, several vaccines, a perspective that makes the anticipation of the vaccine phase complicated, and/or vaccines treating variants). Among the numerous forms of expertise that must be brought into play to manage the coronavirus crisis as best as possible, the human and social sciences must be placed in the front line in order to act on and improve the anticipation and acceptability of anti-epidemic measures.

The second wave, if it is to be confirmed after a lull, will not mark a break from the initial epidemic outbreak, but a continuum, with behaviors inspired by the lessons of the initial phase, dominated by the political desire to manage the social, health and economic problems (these three adjectives could be placed in a different order), with their regional, national and global specificities. As for the third and fourth waves, which are likely, if not certain, they will be associated with a vaccine or vaccines and mass vaccination of more or less anti-vaccine populations, with the major question of (compulsory?) vaccination of health professionals. Finally, another question in terms of anti-vaccination arises: do the specificities of the Covid-19 epidemic prevent us from taking inspiration from the examples of SARS-CoV-1 or the Spanish flu, and thus being one step ahead of the epidemic?

7.3. More questions

First of all, what were, should have been and must be the representations, perceptions, attitudes, initial and future reference points and appropriate behaviors with regard to the Covid-19 pandemic?

How can crisis management actors and decision-makers anticipate, in a context of uncertainty depending on the evolution of a phenomenon that experts (epidemiologists, infectious diseases specialists and scientists dedicated to fundamental research) themselves have difficulty in predicting?

In order to acquire detailed answers to these questions, we need to start, from both a national and international perspective, by analyzing the different strategies implemented over time, from the first weak signals to the return to a quasi-normal situation, which has been characterized by denial and which some associate with vaccination. Faced with the “disruptive pandemic” – that is, SARS-CoV-2, “disruptive” because its possible dynamics are new and unknown – States, even at the European level, have adopted different strategies in terms of screening (serological tests and PCR), prophylaxis (quarantine) and management (transfer of patients). It seems that the guidelines, recommendations and expert opinions are written in a hurry in the current crisis, thereby making it difficult to understand the measures taken, their results and the reactions of the political and health circles and the general public.

In contrast to the “never again” attitude (with particular reference to the First World War and the Spanish flu pandemic of 1918–1919), the exceptional situation created by SARS-CoV-2 requires the anticipation and sharing of all knowledge – some of which, dominated by vaccines, is the property of industrialists – and the adoption of appropriate and rapidly evolving recommendations. Anticipation and the ability to adapt quickly, both individually and collectively, are becoming central in order to implement both top-down (from the State to the individual) and cross-cutting (local, community, interdisciplinary) measures. One of the major problems in this respect is that the knowledge on which to base appropriate decisions is incipient, fragmented and, above all, biased by the diversity of factors to be considered, particularly health, social and economic factors, not to mention the role of media counter-powers (of all kinds).

7.4. From information to communication and education

Communication to the public is increasingly becoming a major societal issue, as is the fight against fake news. A gap exists between the content and evolution of the messages transmitted by decision-makers and the understanding, adherence and (changes in) behavior of the population. This gap is particularly visible through the non-compliance with certain health and social recommendations, and through the constant search for information by the population from all possible sources, including the media and social networks. At any time and on any occasion, the legitimate action of decision-makers through their management of the crisis, starting with that of the State, can be thwarted by media pressure and theatrics. We have seen the rapid and incomprehensible changes in the polls on contamination, the age of people at risk, vaccination, lockdown, etc., all transmitted by the experts and sources of the day.

Two major lessons in this regard concern:

– the place and role of social networks, which are mainly in the hands of Big Tech (Google, Apple, Facebook, Amazon, Microsoft and others);

– the confirmation that medicine is definitely not an exact science if we refer to the perpetual debates between experts.

Another lesson from the health crisis is the uncertainty of the behaviors that must be adopted between generations in order to manage the epidemic in terms of "safety for all": indeed, who is at risk, who is vulnerable and who is a transmitter (in which circumstances, through which social events and which acts of life)? Furthermore, in order to anticipate accurately, it is necessary to highlight the perception of the present and future situation, in terms of understanding and acceptance by various populations, and perceive the logic of action of decision-makers, operational actors and even influencers, such as Professor Didier Raoult. Recommendations based on feedback from home and abroad must be proposed to improve the capacity to respond and help public actors in charge of health and public safety make the right decisions in order to optimize the implementation of anti-epidemic measures in the field.

7.5. Markers of anticipation

What are the pillars of crisis anticipation? At what levels should we act? To be able to anticipate, it seems necessary to:

– Identify and formalize the decision-making dynamics of public authorities and health officials, by integrating national specificities (circulation from the center to the periphery) and their reference systems (scientific committees dominated by experts whose words are more media-oriented than scientific).

– Evaluate the role and impact of multiple sources of information, from mainstream media to social networks and their different types, from experts to word-of-mouth, including micro-influencers.

– Analyze the perceptions of health actors and health professionals, as indispensable representatives in the field, as well as the variety of information and diagnostic tools available (individual dialogue in the office vs. the Web).

– Analyze the perceptions of the general public by all appropriate means, focusing on the emotional and behavioral impact of institutional decisions adopted against Covid-19, and this among the numerous and diverse populations at risk and their personal and professional entourages.

– Evaluate the acceptability and effectiveness of the decisions made, compared with the alternative solutions envisaged in other countries, by contextualizing them in the current situation and uncertainties.

– Provide both a local perspective (fleeing of city dwellers to their second homes in order to be in environments more protected, supposedly, from the epidemic risk) and an international perspective, based on comparisons between the health policy choices made in France, Spain, Italy and Germany.

– Integrate, because of the globalization of information (social networks), the impact of populist and ideological discourses (particularly in the United States, Brazil and China) on the health crisis today and on the vaccine measures tomorrow, which are likely to be as numerous and different as the types, modes of action and expected effects and even side effects of each vaccine produced by industrialists in global competition. In order to anticipate, are the political authorities led, from this perspective, to "secure" the supply of millions of doses?

– Devise, based on a comparative analysis between countries and ideologies, practical tools (decision aids, mementos, methodological guides) and the right media for anticipation and decision-making in order to assess the socio-economic variables and uncertainties that allow for anticipation (alert and emergency phases) and to promote good prevention, protection and communication practices.

In addition to these points, it will be useful to analyze the effects on the behavior of "young people" of communication focused on "vulnerable" people (or those made vulnerable by Covid-19 and possible inappropriate health decisions). For example, did the risks incurred by the elderly and the frail modify the behavior of their (grand)children, who were hardly affected by the epidemic?

7.6. Xth wave

When the time comes, it will also be appropriate to question the semantics used to describe the Covid-19 epidemic. For example, in France, the second epidemic wave has so far been much more similar to the tidal bore (a natural phenomenon in which the water in a river or estuary rises sharply during high tides) at Mont-Saint-Michel than to the monstrous waves at Nazaré, a town on the Atlantic coast of Portugal. How can we convince people about "what is really happening" using a discourse that is based on words that are ambiguous, even bordering on the false, in relation to reality?

Nowhere has a real second wave occurred yet, because there has not been a real global lull, so no one can predict what the behavior of societies will be between the backlash of the (long-awaited) third wave and the "vaccine wave", with the setting up of a competition between States, vaccine laboratories and political decisions.

A final question about the crisis that has shaken and is still shaking the world can be asked as follows: could we have anticipated the social behaviors that arose at the end of the first phase of the Covid-19 epidemic, which in many countries included a laxity in behavior, with a consequent lower respect for sanitary precautions (protective measures, wearing of masks, limitations on socializing)? This laxity is part of the overall societal framework of democratic societies in which respect for freedom can tend to take precedence over all other considerations, particularly those of a health nature.

An emerging topic is *variants*. This is a perfectly normal evolution of a mostly global virus, but new questions, behaviors and radical decisions emerge.

7.7. Conclusion: much remains to be done in the study of behavior related to health crises

Following the current crisis, we must obviously act with reference to the future, but how can we anticipate behaviors and manage them harmoniously?

Action in this field should be organized according to four main types of tasks:

– the collection of scientifically proven knowledge;

– the analysis of the event and decision dynamics;

– the development of a methodological guide and handbook on anticipation and crisis management for decision-makers, influencers and media outlets;

– the development of consistent (for all audiences) and personalized (for each audience) awareness and training.

Finally, the study of behaviors, particularly in relation to compliance with health regulations, is an area of study that should be given greater emphasis, given, on the one hand, the importance of behaviors in the proper management of crises, and on the other hand, the small number of scientific publications on health behaviors (compared, in particular, to the large number of publications on the pathogenic action of SARS-CoV-2 or the preventive and curative treatments of Covid-19). The aim would be to include behavioral experts among the many experts in national committees and health institutions, such as the WHO.

7.8. References

To illustrate the conclusion of this chapter, here is a short list of scientific publications indexed in Medline, the bibliographic database for biomedical sciences, with titles including both the words “Covid-19” and “behavior(al)”.

Ammar, A., Brach, M., Trabelsi, K., Chtourou, H., Boukhris, O., Masmoudi, L., Bouaziz, B., Bentlage, E., How, D., Ahmed, M. et al. (2020). Effects of Covid-19 home confinement on eating behaviour and physical activity: Results of the ECLB-COVID19 international online survey. *Nutrients*, 12(6), 1583.

Clements, J.M. (2020). Knowledge and behaviors toward Covid-19 among US residents during the early days of the pandemic: Cross-sectional online questionnaire. *JMIR Public Health Surveillance*, 6(2), e19161.

Conejero, I., Berrouiguet, S., Ducasse, D. (2020). Suicidal behavior in light of Covid-19 outbreak: Clinical challenges and treatment perspectives. *Encephale*, 46(3S), S66–S72.

Dunton, G.F., Do, B., Wang, S.D. (2020). Early effects of the Covid-19 pandemic on physical activity and sedentary behavior in children living in the U.S. *BMC Public Health*, 20(1), 1351.

Hall, G., Laddu, D.R., Phillips, S.A., Lavie, C.J., Arena, R. (2020). A tale of two pandemics: How will Covid-19 and global trends in physical inactivity and sedentary behavior affect one another? *Progress in Cardiovascular Diseases*, 8 April.

Hansel, T.C. and Saltzman, L.Y. (2020). Behavioral health and response for Covid-19. *Disaster Medicine and Public Health Preparedness*, 29, 1–7.

Jiao, W.Y., Wang, L.N., Liu, J., Fang, S.F., Jiao, F.Y., Pettoello-Mantovani, M., Somekh, E. (2020). Behavioral and emotional disorders in children during the Covid-19 epidemic. *Journal of Pediatrics*, 221, 264–266.

López-Bueno, R., Calatayud, J., Casaña, J., Casajus, J.A., Smith, L., Tully, M.A., Andersen L.L., Lopez-Sanchez, G.F. (2020). Covid-19 confinement and health risk behaviors in Spain. *Frontiers in Psychology*, 11, 1426.

Ortmann, R., Pelster, M., Wengerek, S.T. (2020). Covid-19 and investor behavior. *Finance Research Letters*, 8 August, 101717.

8

Humans, Digital Technology and the SARS-CoV-2 Health Crisis

The human factor is the term by which specialists in the field of human safety and plant security refer to the behavior of people at work. This "factor" is frequently invoked in the analysis of industrial disasters, industrial accidents, and in court cases or commissions of inquiry, and is generally associated with the idea of fault. Paradoxically, this negative conception of human intervention is based on an unquestioning confidence in technology and on a lack of knowledge of the human sciences.

Dejours (2014, p. 48)

8.1. Introduction

Have you noticed how quickly our behaviors have changed in connection with the communication around the health crisis? Similarly, did you notice a "transformation" in our humanity, sociality and social emotions? As we went out, little by little, in the lockdown period, which started in March 2020, did you also experience the change in relation to the *Homo sapiens* dress code, with the compulsory wearing of the mask – despite its lack of availability – a bottle of hand sanitizer, gloves (equally contradictory recommendations followed each other on this subject) and a visor. Or, again, did you experience the new rules of social distancing – through the respect of a distance of one meter, or even two, between individuals, that is, a great distance at first sight – and, since the easing of restrictions, those of house

Chapter written by Judith NICOGOSSIAN.

arrest, the passage to sanitary instructions, sometimes understandable, sometimes abstruse, and so on. In the way of greeting each other? Of saying hello to a loved one? To kiss or not to kiss, such has become the question asked at every friendly meeting. Generally, the question is whether we prefer to respect the instructions or whether we decide to kiss each other against all odds. The mask standard has been imposed, and people who are not masked up may be refused access to a place; in this game of masks, you might as well have one in your pocket, regardless of its actual quality. It is not uncommon to see two masked people who decide to lift their masks to get along better or to see each other smile, or for some other reason. Today masks are lying around, crumpled up in the bottom of a handbag; they are exchanged, lent, purchased at the last minute, with a range of prices depending on the goodwill of shopkeepers. The effective lack of mask hygiene questions its real antiviral properties, while the wearing of the mask on the face questions the felt loneliness of the fields of masked faces. The health recommendations of wearing a mask have transformed emotional and sensory communication – with the mask, we can no longer see our mouths, our smiles, we hear each other less well, words are muffled; thanks to wearing a mask, we have realized that we also lip read. A large number of the micro-movements of the face are no longer perceptible and we plunge into a form of anonymity. When we put the FFP2 mask on our face before entering a shop, we have the strange feeling of organizing a hold-up. This crisis has brutally confronted us with an impoverishment of human contact, and it has radicalized the *absence of contact* and established a regime of distance. Have you noticed how, in the few weeks following the declaration of the health crisis, the simple fact of crossing a passer-by on a pavement became complicated, even unpleasant? In Spain, pedestrians, for fear of crossing other passers-by on the pavement, prefer to walk on the road, which is a source of accidents. Have you noticed regional, national, European and international disparities in health crisis management – such as between France and a very close country, Germany? Cognitive dissonance? Orders and counter-orders? Have you also noticed the existence of insoluble contradictions between doctors and politicians, and between the saying and doing of communication? Have you noticed the therapeutic confusion of knowledge and practices, of remedies and poisons, of conventional medicine? Finally, have you noticed the anxiety-inducing media entropy of our information and communication society?

Through the health crisis, humans found themselves at fault, presumed guilty of circulating the virus, precisely that of Covid-19, and of being contagious. On this accusation, *sapiens* were therefore asked to stop their contacts. The mask became an exo-organ with a prophylactic effect, much like the statues of the saints in the churches of the Middle Ages. The solutions to the crisis eventually appeared to depend on remote communication technologies. However, given the negative conception of human intervention that emerged – via our latent fault of being able to fall ill or contaminate others – we relied on an unquestioning trust in technology, and on a blatant ignorance of the human sciences. Do we need to be reminded of the intrinsic properties of the species, both on the biological level and on the closely related level of our cultures, our practices and our traditions? How can we adapt, in this context of health crisis, to the systematic use of remote communication tools?

Communication in the context of a health crisis has borrowed clichés; it has brought about many contradictory injunctions, misunderstandings, cognitive dissonances, a false binarity between reason and emotion, a radicalization of technologies; and it has had the particularity of provoking breaking points in the physical body. Poor communication on health has acted like a collective nocebo, plunging us into a total misunderstanding of the situation. Today, out of house arrest, most of us have spent a wisely touristy summer, with a majority of people having boycotted the airports; many stayed at home. We have gradually fallen into the discomfort of a conditional freedom whose limits are those of the other's body, or worse, of our own body. We have become the object of a certain traceability, at least in intention. According to certain socio-professional categories, we must follow demanding sanitary protocols. The French government is imposing data traceability measures, an undertaking that will be blatantly unsuccessful because the data war has already (too) long given primacy to digital sovereignty, the pace of which is set in the West by Big Tech (Google, Amazon, Facebook, Microsoft, IBM). Whether we are aware of it or not, these measures sow confusion, stress and friction by presenting the necessary conditions of a windfall for the control companies.

It is clear that, even in good health, we physically feel the effects of communication about the virus. From the very beginning of the decision to confine people, a notion of apprehension, not to say *fear* – feaer of contagion, of going out, of touching, of being in the way – or of shame is established as soon as one of the many potential clinical signs of Covid-19 appears, such as a cold, a cough or temporary fatigue. In this era of health doubt and relentless standardization, there has been a great confusion of meaning. For example, even in the midst of good health, we have each surprised ourselves by thinking ourselves asymptomatic, turning ourselves in to a feeling reminiscent of Jules Romain's self-evident truth.

8.2. Physical and digital communication in a crisis situation

What is new compared to previous epidemics, such as the Hong Kong flu in 1968–1970 (31,000 victims in France), is that in 2020, information and communication technologies allowed us to communicate remotely, which is of great importance in a context of total confinement of populations.

These tools question the transferability of the physical relationship to the digital relationship. Lockdown and quarantine measures related to the pandemic cut us off from the physical world, making us avoid points of contact, which have become points of contagion, through a sudden semantic shift.

One way to overcome isolation is to get connected, provided that the right technologies are available. Lockdown has led to an impressive acceleration in digital transformation in the field of health[1], for example through telemedicine, and also in other areas, such as education and work.

Complementary to physical communication, the experience of lockdown has exceptionally accelerated the shift to digital communication, dematerializing encounters. We are experiencing this dematerialization for better or worse – for better, because without it we could not "keep" ourselves locked up without contact; and for worse, because some people have suffered an impoverishment of the therapeutic relationship with their medical contacts because of tele-distancing. Thus, 20 million chronically ill people, people in rehabilitation, cancer patients and people waiting for surgery or dental care, as well as the elderly, have been left without contact.

There are many reasons for these dysfunctions, either relating to the inadequacy of health regulations for the crisis situation or to the lack of organization and the unpreparedness of those involved in remote care. These reasons do not necessarily depend on a feeling of the impoverished quality of virtual exchanges (although remoteness has sacrificed the sense of touch, reduced motivation and dealt a blow to pedagogy). While there are benefits

1 The crisis situation has boosted medical teleconsultation (Sanofi Lab Santé 2020).

to be credited to lockdown, such as a reorganization of our lifestyles and our way of consuming and producing and, moreover, helping in the fight against global warming, we already see many dysfunctions linked to this situation. We must therefore look into the analysis of the experimentation that has been the lockdown period, and evaluate it through feedback, in order to design a future that remains desirable.

How can we use remote communication tools in the service of a health crisis? What would be the *good uses* with regard to the health of the "remotely communicating" body?

The richness of the human experiment that was lockdown is equal to its failures, with the question that is the focus in this matter thus becoming: to what extent can the digital world represent the physical world with regard to the care pathways? How can we think about the hybridization of the screen and the human being in the context of social ties? How can we continue to evolve in an environment that has to take into account data from the organic world and data from the electronic world through the neologism that marketing has proposed, a term that is somewhat devoid of meaning, the "phygital"?

8.3. A little reminder about communication

Anthropology, behavioral sciences, medicine, psychiatry, neuroscience – each of these disciplines has contributed to the fascinating observation of human communication over more than a century.

For the Palo Alto school of thought, it appears that we use two modes of communication – verbal and non-verbal[2]:

– *Verbal* communication is said to be "digital"[3]: the explicit meaning is carried by words, allowing the use of words to build a logical and precise

---

2 Albert Merhabian, a psychologist, stated the "3 Vs" rule, which corresponds to the fact that only 7% of communication is carried out using the meaning of words, while 38% is vocal, using intonation and the sound of the voice, and 55% is visual, using facial expressions and body language (Mehrabian et al. 1967).

3 The father of communication anthropology, Gregory Bateson, from the Palo Alto school of thought, referred to "digital" verbal communication. The term "digital" comes from the Latin *digitus*, which means "finger"; "digit" means a number (0 to 9). It has been used with regard to computing since 1945. In 1964, the French *l'Histoire générale des sciences* presented "the

discourse, and the analysis of what is said. This form of communication explains and interprets through the use of verbal codes and is formatted by language codes. In order to communicate, it is necessary for individuals to have a common meaning.

– *Non-verbal* communication is known as "analogical": the meaning is outside the words, in sounds, movement, the look, touch, intonation; that is, it is affective, more vague and uses symbols (tone, intonation, the look, body expression, dress code). This communication is immediately understood by all, universally; it is supposedly more intuitive, as it is based on instinctive behaviors[4].

Today, thanks to the Internet, a third mode of communication has emerged. Through the Web, the known limits of time and space are transcended. The use of remote technologies, which no longer require the physical presence of two or more protagonists in an exchange, in fact modifies the intrinsic properties of human communication (both verbal and non-verbal). This third mode of communication implies the production and provision of human–machine interaction technologies. From an anthropobiological point of view, this other mode of communication can be described as "phygital" (situated between the physical and digital body) because it brings the human body into a new paradigm.

8.3.1. *Use case: the Covid-19 health crisis*

Understanding the strategy of the SARS-CoV-2 virus is a major challenge in controlling the spread of the epidemic and developing

---

history of so-called digital machines". "Digital", in English, is specific to computer processing, without the ambiguity that "*numérique*" has in French between its mathematical and statistical use and its application to computers. Subject to fashions, variations and communication strategies, French hesitates between "*numérique*" and "*digital*". In French, "digital" is first and foremost what is related to fingers. The official French and Quebec terminologies prefer "*numérique*", yet the use of "*digital*" in French continues as a synonym. The context guides in cases of ambiguity. Except in a humorous way, "*empreinte digitale*" (digital footprint) is not synonymous with "*empreinte numérique*".

4 Metacommunication is understood to be a special form of communication that indicates how verbal information should be interpreted, taking into account non-verbal stimuli seen as metacommunicative signals that can reinforce or contradict verbal information. This reciprocal influence of messages in a synergistic combination is a function of communication, which can be verbal or non-verbal.

therapeutic knowledge (Elsevier 2020), including a vaccine (WHO 2020). The Covid-19 virus is biological; however, it is also the object of a scientific and cultural construction. French society's major fear about the virus has focused on the capacity to care for patients in hospitals and on the availability of the necessary medical equipment, which may in fact be lacking.

The communication about the virus – and the political decision to lock down the population – generated a response in terms of behavior with a real impact on the organization of life. The *narrative* conveyed through the virus functioned as a prompter, that is, as a driving force of behavior. This narrative was constructed both in terms of reason and in terms of emotions. The arrival of the virus led to the implementation of a national strategy, with health laws such as quarantining and the wearing of masks, which upset social organization and changed customs, rituals and practices.

However, if each person invests their own flows of desires and beliefs in the narrative machine, there always remains a part of freedom in the human being (Citton 2010). Thus, our communication is at the service of value systems that oppose and confront each other, with the construction of reality and behavior at stake, and along with the definition of what the human being should be in a given society, and what our bodies, uses and rituals, health, illness and care should be in particular.

For Claude Lévi-Strauss, the true function of a myth – such as that of the construction of behaviors in the face of the virus – is to "provide a logical model capable of overcoming a contradiction (an unattainable task, when the contradiction is real)" (Lévi Strauss 1962, 1973). The regulation that has been put in place raises questions about crisis management, during and also after the crisis, as well as the impact of its consequences and our future. The health crisis situation speaks of our relationship with the virus, disease, death and our knowledge; however, it also implies that we cannot dissociate our lives from the general organization of the living.

8.3.2. *Worrying?*

> It's completely unprecedented, we're not prepared! – Julie, 21 (Nicogossian 2020).

For the historian Faure, "there is no reason to say that, with the SARS-CoV-2 epidemic, France is now experiencing the greatest health crisis in its history, unless we start the story in 1960" (Faure 2020). Smallpox, for its part, wreaked havoc from the Neolithic period until it was completely eradicated in the 20th century thanks to vaccination campaigns. In 1349, the bubonic plague decimated a quarter of the European population; in the 20th century, starting in 1918, the Spanish flu (subtype H1N1 of influenza A) killed between 17 and 100 million people. Then, in 1968, the Hong Kong flu (subtype H3N2 of influenza A) killed 1 million people worldwide.

The political thought of the 21st century constructs its discourse by moving away from Darwin and the principle of survival, in nature of *the fittest*. It is this paradigm shift that gives Covid-19 the status of "the greatest health crisis in history". Yet, although we are not just discovering the virus or the lockdown situation – or even death – it is more difficult to accept in the 21st century that the virus can kill[5]. The state is establishing an anti-historical discourse on a death principle as unacceptable. This discourse reflects the paradigm shift in health care, but can be seen as historically misleading[6].

Similarly, the number of deaths attributed to Covid-19 is consistent with the usual number of deaths linked to winter flu episodes each year (290,000 to 650,000 deaths per year worldwide). This figure is of little significance (even though we must pay tribute to the victims of the pandemic) when compared to other problems, such as those resulting from industrial practices; for example, air pollution is estimated to cause nine million deaths per year worldwide, including 67,000 in France; as for smoking, in 2015 it caused "only" 7.2 million deaths worldwide.

From the perspective of a prioritization of health hazards at the global level, Covid-19 is not a main issue, while access to water is crucial: by 2025, 50% of the world's population will indeed live in areas of diminished access to and/or quality of drinking water (OMS 2019). Undernourishment is also of greater concern than Covid-19, with 821 million people worldwide suffering from hunger, or one in nine people (WFP 2019):

---

5 The ideology of technological progress, embodied by transhumanism, considers death as a disease (JIM 2020).

6 To date, the SARS-CoV-2 coronavirus has caused nearly 31,000 deaths in France; this is obviously 31,000 deaths too many; however, it should be noted that these deaths represent a little over 5% of the 580,000 annual deaths in France (Worldometers 2020).

> A world whose population I have seen increase sixfold appears to me to be hopeless (Levi-Strauss 2004).

In our collective imagination, we would rather suffer from a situation of overpopulation and depletion of resources (Worldometers 2020), than from a scenario of collapse of the human species. As an indication, our planet welcomes some 200,000 new individuals every day. We would rather be facing the opposite problem of a vertiginous demographic explosion. Thus, apologizing for the insensitivity of his analysis, Emmanuel Todd indicated that "the vitality of a society is measured more by its capacity to give birth than by its capacity to save its elderly" (Chartier 2020).

8.4. Living and the organization of life

The story of the "new coronavirus", which began in Wuhan, is an episode in humanity's fight against disease and the postponement of death.

Ancient Greece was the scene of a civilization that saw the birth of great physicians and which described life using two different terms:

– *zoe*, which is the fact of living, not distinguishing us from other animals or plants;

– *bios*, which is the way of life, the cultural construction of life that politics contributes to taking care of.

"Being alive" is therefore a matter of *zoe*, whereas lockdown measures are a matter of organizing life, that is, *bios*. In 2020, unlike in ancient Greece, politics took charge of our health at the level of *bios*, but also of *zoe*, which corresponds to the health care we know in societies today. For the state, the individual is considered as a healthy body, while for the individual, good health is considered as a given.

8.5. Different value systems in conflict

8.5.1. *Reason and emotion (between individual and person)*

The "human factor" has an inescapable place in the event of a crisis, because humans are the heart of crises and their management process. The communication of the Covid-19 health crisis led to controversies about a set of definitions, those of the scientist, the carer and care, and opposed several belief systems, that of political discourse versus that of practicing medicine and health versus regulations. Communication on the virus, conveyed by language, has been the subject of a formatting of meaning, which a set of actors has relayed, at the national or international level, through politicians, journalists and every one of us:

> In a crisis, the different sectors, with both the actors who traditionally drive them, and the norms that routinely govern them, collude and interpenetrate (Dobry 1986).

For Dobry, the de-sectorization of the social space supporting this observation has two components: the reduction of autonomy, which may correspond to a source of divergence between the actors involved, who, if they perceive that their autonomy is reduced for the benefit of the other actors will not get involved in the interrelated system; and, in contrast, the de-sectorization of the spaces of confrontation, "the idea being then that the issues of the crisis are themselves difficult to define and master, and that there is a competition for this very definition" (Boumrar and Bordes 2015). The difficulty lies in the fact of a permanent confrontation of value systems that oppose and clash.

The first component, that of the lack of involvement of certain actors due to a reduction of their autonomy, is perfectly illustrated by the Covid-19 health crisis. The emergence of the carer, valued, hyper-solicited and widely manipulated by politicians and the media, was actively involved in the management of the crisis. The main problem with the figure of the *hero* is that it is constituted in opposition to other "deactivated" individuals, passive objects of care. The extent of the impact of this phenomenon has begun to be seen in some of the reactions of other socio-professional categories to reduced lockdown measures (e.g. the "deactivated" figure comprised by an impressive group of elementary and high school teachers, who suddenly did not want to return to their educational activities). The capacitated construction of the figure of the carer – as a hero – was inscribed in the symbolism of a movement from the individual to the collective. The soft incentives (nudges) and injunctions in the construction of the figure of the carer as the hero of this health war, carried by the political discourse and conveyed by the media, soon came into play in the collective imagination of the population. The carers (as individuals), towards whom all our attention has converged, have been admired for their dedication and their remarkable adaptive capacity (e.g. the redeployment of some of them in hospitals) which has encouraged acts of bravery on a collective and individual scale. However, this construction has also weakened the other categories of the population, which have become very vulnerable, isolated and passive, as in the case of the inadequate care of the sick who are left to fend for themselves at home.

Nevertheless, carers (as people) are not disembodied heroes fashioned, in the image of a time of war, with a great deal of lyrical narcissism; they do not survive on the love of caring actions and they are also exposed to illness, subject to negative emotions (Noël 2020) and have material needs.

The second component, that of confusion linked to the competition of the stakes of the crisis, was perfectly illustrated in the conflict between reason and emotion in reference to the definition of the "good scientist". A communication from the French National Scientific Research Center (*Centre national de la recherche scientifique*, CNRS) reminded us, during the epidemic period, of what a scientific message should be in a health crisis situation, following, between passion and reason, a precise code of ethics (Ganascia 2020).

Through the CNRS press release, we understand that the scientist's ethics must in principle be based on a principle of reason. Indeed, reason – necessary for the organization of collective life – is governed by language codes ("a formatting of meaning"), the learning of a methodology and the respect of a regulation. Reason implies that the speaker needs to spend enough time thinking about what they are saying and constructing their demonstration. In terms of reception, the meaning formatted in the sense of reason is then received by the addressee of the message, leaving no room for emotion and inducing an ethical value for the scientific message, in terms of pure truth.

Emotion, which a person is prey to instinctively, is a matter of intuitive communication, and this as opposed to reason, which implies that giving in to "passion" and making decisions without weighing the consequences is conduct unworthy of the scientific approach. This posture defending a scientist's ethics is intelligible in terms of the political question linked to health crisis management, which ultimately still aims to find a happy medium between the principle of collectivity – the unit of which is the individual – and its counterpart, the person (their feelings). Nevertheless, this posture becomes problematic because it also implies that we can access a scientific reason or truth, whereas there are as many types of reason as there are visions in science, and they generally complement and contradict each other. Access to any scientific truth is, moreover, "the nightmare of machine learning" because learning all published scientific texts does not allow for the acquisition of a truthful discourse on a question. The "lack of truth" in statistics, in connection with its many interpretation biases, is well echoed by Mark Twain's adage that "there are three kinds of lies: lies, damned lies and statistics". This posture is also surprising because it implies that we oppose reason and emotion, which is criticizable with regard to our scientific knowledge; we know indeed that the sample of our emotions helps guide our adaptive choices (our actions). Some of our decisions, between what we can explain and what we cannot explain, are instinctual. We cannot, in any domain, separate the reason system (the learned one) from the emotional system (the instinct one) (Verweij et al. 2015). Our scientific principles – scientific truth and the construction of its object – are based on a Cartesian historicist approach, which is widely criticized as reductionist positivism. Thus, the system of acquired methods of scientific validation, and its methodological criteria of veracity, has been opposed, in the context of the Covid-19 crisis, to the principle of a field science appearing to act, in its singular and experimental approach, outside the regulatory framework.

8.5.2. *Governance by affect*

Emotions play a fundamental role in the adaptation of living beings to the environment. Without feeling emotion, we would be unable to make adaptive choices (MIT 2014). Similarly, political communication does not only operate on the register of reason, but also nests in a principle of "affective governance" (Illouz 2006) in which affects are solicited in the expected modification of behavior.

8.5.3. *Laughter*

We universally use a register – a mix of emotions – to guide us and choose our actions, such as courage, frustration, a feeling of being left out leading to demotivation, laughter or fear.

To combat the fear of the health crisis and the alienation associated with its restrictions, such as lockdown, many humorous videos circulated on the Internet. Laughter and derision were an important outlet during the anxiety-inducing lockdown period. One example was a hilarious video of an Italian man toasting his reflection in his bathroom mirror and saying, "thank you for coming!" (New York Times 2020), voted the funniest man alive. Everyone contributes to this digital momentum of exchange, in a lockdown period, thanks to chronicles of the event, for example *1001 Nights of the Wuhan Flue* (Warner 2020). These moments of humor, which are very rich and life-saving, have served their purpose: to alleviate the idleness and the feeling of powerlessness and help endure the confusion.

8.5.4. *Fear*

The political discourse played on the negative emotion of fear. The virus was presented as a single-celled blob, spread over the Earth, aiming to invade and wipe it out. Worthy of an invasion of malicious parasites from a horror movie, making *Alien* look almost cheap, our Covid-19 virus did not just screw up a single spaceship. It gradually spread across the globe, moving from one country to another. Then, it incarnated itself more insidiously, on the mouth of the loved one, coughing; on the postman's shirt, handing us the mail; on a door handle; on an intercom button; behind a neighbor's mask; in the babbling of a 3-year-old child; on a policeman's pen – who, by the way, constrained my 78- and 82-year-old parents for a baguette purchase, because it was forbidden to be out in twos during the lockdown.

The construction of verbal, non-verbal and metacommunication discourse pressed the fear button and served as the grounds for the rise in negative emotions. What has Covid-19 done to us, or rather what has its construction done to us? The consequences of crisis communication generate a confusion of feelings that, in contrast to laughter, often reveal the fragile exterior of our societal humanity:

> Personally, it didn't change me too much, because with my wife I was already confined for 14 years. On the other hand, to have it happen 10 days after our separation, well, I really feel like I'm being punished, that I did something wrong in another life – Vincent, 44 (Nicogossian 2020).

The "fear of contamination" organizes a tension in collective and individual imaginations and justifies many biases in behavior. Thus, the "migration" of Parisians to their second homes in the provinces became a target for denunciation by year-round residents, who were prey to a rise in intolerance and surprising reactions, such as the desire to be checked, in order to reassure themselves. It was also surprising to see the lack of solidarity between different countries on a European scale, and also between different regions and territories within the same country:

> You can see that they are there, the Parisians, as if by chance all the second homes are occupied. They don't respect anything. Nobody tells them anything! Even I haven't been checked yet! – Jeanne, 51 (Nicogossian 2020).

French-style lockdown, surprisingly based on a Chinese-style model – what would Mao do? – had the characteristic of losing people by stressing them violently between action, enaction and inaction, with effects that provoked worry through a rise in anti-democratic and/or anti-humanist impulses. It was a strange feeling, sometimes, to find oneself in the first chapter of a book by Aldous Huxley! Yet, if we follow the philosopher Comte Sponville, "is not catching Covid-19 really a sufficient goal in existence?" (France inter 2020).

The emotion of fear generates unfortunate effects on human behavior, such as a rise in extremist attitudes and rejection of others: withdrawal, alienation, the flip side of the ingredients of a great civilization. Is it necessary to recall Roosevelt's quotation: "So, first of all, let me assert my firm belief that the only thing we have to fear is... fear itself – nameless, unreasoning, unjustified terror which paralyzes needed efforts to convert retreat into advance" (Roosevelt 1933). The questioning of being able to avoid resorting to fear is addressed to politics, to the point of questioning the very definition of health: is *fear* an ingredient of a strong society, is it compatible with good health, the right decisions, the feeling of being well cared for?

Fear and punitive confinement appear to be vectors of degradation of social bonds, hindering the elementary principles of mutual aid and solidarity. Alex Kahn, president of the *Ligue contre le cancer*, reminds us in his position against partial easing of lockdown – evoked for a moment by the state – that 80–85% of volunteers are retired (Kahn 2020). Partial easing of restrictions would have meant "releasing" only healthy people and young people, but not the elderly and those considered vulnerable. Alex Kahn finally recalled an important societal principle, quite fundamental, that consists of bringing help to others, in particular through voluntary work, which is mainly led by the elderly and is a strong vector of social bonds.

Would it not have been wiser to have built a narrative involving courage around the epidemic, which would have solicited the health "helpers" when visiting the neighborhood, instead of each person isolating in fear and passivity? We could have imagined a system of electronic micro-training sessions to encourage everyone to learn techniques likely to help those around them, rather than shutting themselves off.

This system would have had the advantages of:

– *alleviating* the workload of health care professionals;

– *reassuring* people isolating (sick or in good health);

– *enhancing the value* of people who were unemployed thanks to solidarity action;

– *reducing* the negative health effects associated with lockdown;

– *addressing* issues that give *meaning* to our lives;

– *maintaining* social bonds;

– *coordinating* (equally) the actions of the digital and the physical.

8.6. French communication on the virus

Was it the fear of protest that led politicians to adopt health measures unprecedented in history, that is, to completely lock down a countries? Politicians had to encounter the dual challenge of having to deal with the material constraints of the French health system and maximizing its efficiency by managing the risk of a pandemic. Between these two constraints, the progressive implementation of strict rules was the subject of a communication plan that was sometimes incomprehensible (municipal elections maintained at the beginning of the pandemic, total lockdown, supply of masks from China, etc.).

The question of the choice of lockdown on a national scale arose in comparison with other legislation, such as that of the neighboring country, Germany. The refusal of generalized lockdown in France, accompanied by the adoption of reassuring terms, was based on the assumed priority of not worrying the population.

Germany was able to exercise this choice of mass screening versus arbitrary and total lockdown thanks to a capacity to carry out a large number of locally produced tests; in terms of health prevention, the adoption of measures quarantining only vulnerable populations or those at particular risk of contamination was sufficient. As for the reactivity of health industrialists, such as Sanofi, it allowed, prior to the development of a vaccine, the free and immediate provision of 100 million doses of hydroxychloroquine to the governments of many countries, while at the same time dedicating European production means to a future vaccine.

The two leaders, Angela Merkel for Germany and Emmanuel Macron for France, did not have the same approach to the crisis. Indeed, “Germany is not France, we don’t have a President at war, we have a Chancellor who is quite calm, who measures her words, who acts in tandem with her government and the Länder” (Vasak 2020)[7].

8.6.1. *Myth of war*

For Yves Citton, these are “the narrative pre-scripted behaviors”. Thus, when unexpected events occur, behavior is based on everything that feeds memory. The official narrative is then put at the service of a kind of *mythocracy* (Citton 2010), which is of the order of the imaginary and develops according to three issues: the modeling of a theory of power based on the circulation of narratives, the concept of scripting and the demonstration that scripting is not necessarily negative.

Thus, the use of the semantic field of war (“*state of siege*”), and the circulation of soldiers in the cities, probably encouraged citizens to raid the shops – to stock up on pasta, rice, sugar and flour – by reintroducing in people’s minds an *imaginary* wartime including food shortages, and similarly, the figure of the hero came to reinforce this idea of war and induced the putting forward of the notion of sacrifice:

> I have enough to last for six months at home. You never know
> – Antoine, 71 (Nicogossian 2020).

7 Henrik Uterwedde, researcher at the Franco-German Institute in Ludwigsburg, interviewed by the radio station France Culture.

The meaning of words and the definitions of terms are important in terms of how a message is received. For example, the term "lockdown" itself is probably inappropriate, as it sounds like a punitive measure, whereas there is no intention to damage *social bonds* through it. As some studies have (already) shown, this situation of social isolation is psychologically *violent* and causes brain damage (Tomova et al. 2020). For the neuropsychiatrist Boris Cyrulnik, the term "crisis" used in relation to Covid-19 was also ill-chosen, as it is a medical term whose etymology is linked to the manifestation of a disease. In his view, the term "catastrophe" was more appropriate, because "a star is going out" and we are "experiencing a huge assault, which we are dealing with as best we can". In this sense, many doctors are concerned about the collateral effects of lockdown on the health of a representative part of the population ("when life returns, it will not be the same") (Cyrulnik 2020). This life now "in danger", faced with an idea of death that has become omnipresent, is embodied by Covid-19. The personification of death concretized by the outbreak of the coronavirus served to operate a change of operational behavior, corresponding to the fact of focusing henceforth on the fear of dying due to Covid-19 (a way of supplanting the other health risks) and of assimilating Covid-19 to physical contact, and thus of eliminating any form of physical contact to eliminate contagion, and even of sacrificing the content of the social bond to overcome death.

All practices and representations of "touch" (Vinit et al. 2006) have been affected by the crisis. Medical, anthropological and philosophical knowledge is unanimous: *the skin is an essential organ*, because it allows us to feel and open our body to the world, and touch is of primary importance for well-being and health[8]. Skin and touch are intrinsic properties of our species that cannot be reduced to a vector of contamination (let us recall, via the knowledge acquired about *microbiota*, that we permanently host 2 to 3 kilograms of foreign hosts in our digestive tract, mainly bacteria, yeasts, fungi and viruses, and that we are not bubble beings endowed with an aseptic environment, but living homeostasis beings in a permanent process of rebalancing with our biological and climatic environment).

A double bind presented conflicting information that had the effect of raising the stress level of individuals, notably through the *dressing code of*

8 Pirrko Routasalo proposes a typology of touch according to five types: technical, communicational, relational, therapeutic and energetic (Routasalo 1999).

the new soldier, who was then, through the mouth of the French president, going to war naked. Thus, the panoply included:

– masks, which had to be worn, but which were not or only partially available, and moreover not very or only partially effective (especially in view of the real uses made of them);

– tests, which were not available, were not produced locally and had to wait for delivery from China;

– disinfectant gel, the composition of which is not necessarily suitable for health and skin;

– resuscitation beds, the number of which had been reduced and whose shortage had to be made up for urgently, without the decisions that led to the reduction being denounced.

Will the anxiety-provoking constructs surrounding the SARS-CoV-2 crisis cause more irreparable damage to living beings than the virus itself? The orchestration of the symbolic order implies, as we know, the physical control of the population. Nevertheless, in terms of the mind, of the biological body, the violence linked to lockdown has been significant and, if we risk a minimum of slight stress, a maximum of "atrophy" of cerebral plasticity is nonetheless at stake, depending on the resilience capacity of people in managing the crisis they are confronted with (Cyrulnik 2020).

> Shopping; and then eating is the only thing I have left. All my volunteer activities have stopped. I'm bored and feel like I'm useless. – Mrs. Vale, 67 (Nicogossian 2020).

8.6.2. *Sensemaking*

The notion of *sensemaking* corresponds to the meaning that individuals give to what they do. In this context, one of the roles of the societal organization is to help give meaning to the activities of individuals. In a crisis situation, it is a matter of being interested in the way human beings, through what they do in society, give meaning to their actions (Weick 1988). Indeed, actors act more logically if they know how to act and if a formalized crisis management process seems to have positive effects on the crisis they are facing. The notion of creativity is a societal process of joint evolution of collective actions intertwined with the interpretations of individuals

(Magakian 2006), at the intersection of individual and collective action. The positive virtues of creativity on the "morale of the troops" could be observed in France through the solidarity and home-made manufacture of "protective masks" during the health crisis, according to a manufacturing standard proposed for the occasion (Afnor 2020), and through the intermediary of mask-making tutorials that were taken up by an entire country.

The (European) countries managed the health crisis in different ways, which is somewhat paradoxical given that it respnded to a common biological hazard that knows no borders. It should have been possible to explain the European health crisis rationally, in *a reasoned manner* and in real time, for example on a dedicated television channel. Coherent communication has only advantages, as it builds confidence in the solutions adopted and allows the public to support the solutions adopted. For example, a principle of solidarity encouraged by a community of caregivers or volunteers would have made it possible to: create meaning before the loosening of restrictions; install mutual aid mechanisms in the face of real needs; boost the acquisition and transmission of useful techniques; and mitigate the effects of social isolation.

8.6.3. *Importance of rituals*

> Since the lockdown, I eat well: I go and buy fresh products every day, to have a bit of color on my plate. But I miss my life before lockdown: in the morning I used to drink my coffee on the terrace at Jussieu, and then often for my lunch break, I went to the Jardin des Plantes. Once a week, I went to see a movie at the Art Cinema. After almost 2 months, I feel depressed. I work less well remotely. I keep doing webinars. I can't take it anymore. I miss everything – Ivan, 43 (Nicogossian 2020).

Rituals are founding elements of our humanity, of our social organization, of which we do not yet understand the full importance in terms of the brain; for example, of the emotions necessary for social cohesion, such as well-being and empathy.

The anthropologist Fabienne Martin-Juchat raises the question of the rituals of politeness associated with the physical world, which are emblematic of sociality and are of great importance. These rituals have a function that we lose in practices carried out remotely: that of avoiding the feeling of aggression generated by co-presence (Martin-Juchat 2020) by giving us a feeling of well-being, involving a hormonal release, such as serotonin or oxytocin in the body, which we associate with happiness. We have experienced the fact fact of isolating ourselves, of being socially cut off from each other, of no longer frequenting our favorite places – restaurants, bars, parties and concerts – of no longer visiting our family, our friends; of being cut off from our micro-rituals, love, work, meetings, our bodily behaviors, our street activities, our impressions, our expressions, such as no longer greeting, or being greeted behind a mask; of being cut off from our founding beliefs, some of our values, religious meetings, such as the forbidden and/or limited access to the funerals of our loved ones. All these shortages and impossibilities induce, beyond the production of negative emotions and a state of depression, a phenomenon of brutal *deculturation*, which can be seen as the paradoxical flip side of a policy of "care taking".

8.7. Healing (medicine) and caring (attention)

Health professionals, men and women in the field, must respond to an emergency situation. They provide technical care, medication (a cure) and also an *emotional principle*, attention (care) responding to the immediate needs of the sick.

In the management of the health crisis that we have just experienced, we have seen that reason and passion confront each other. This opposition can be illustrated in the difference between cure and care, between *curing as medicine* and *caring as attention* given to the sick person. Although curing and caring should ideally be complementary in therapeutic terms, the debate in fact opposes two value systems. The cure system embodies the collective of the political and/or regulatory order, where the individual takes precedence over the person; and the care system embodies the caregiver in the field who has to manage emergency situations when faced with a patient waiting for an immediate solution, prioritizing imperatives based on the person's feelings. On this subject, we have seen that a field care situation located in the middle of a "health crisis" prioritizes caring and curing in equal measure.

8.8. People and the Internet: from physical to digital

Information and communication technologies, such as the Internet, have taken on a major role in the new situation that is being played out through the dissemination of government information, both nationally and internationally; the responsiveness expected of citizens; and finally, the way in which citizen-users are make use of these tools.

Remote control technologies have made it possible to relay certain social rituals through new *techniques* developed by their users. For example, the *Orchestre National de France* (French National Orchestra) proposed a dystopian performance full of poetry in a remote interpretation of Ravel's Bolero, where the engineer edited the various pieces as much as a musician, certainly replacing the conductor of the physical world (France Musique 2020), but whose actors actively contributed to the positive emotional enrichment of digital communication. More generally, the practice of webinars has largely inaugurated another way of organizing conferences and meetings that bring together different actors remotely around a theme. Similarly, telemedicine has taken over from physical consultations in doctors' offices or hospitals when therapeutic advice is given to patients.

However, it was necessary to learn very quickly how to surf the Internet during the crisis because, in order to awaken to the meaning of the "phygital", it was necessary to manage the coming and going of the flow of information and to protect oneself from it – which is not obvious in the absence of dedicated training (it is not enough, in fact, to have a connected screen for remote management to work and for the message to make sense to its recipient).

8.8.1. *Infobesity*

According to Umberto Eco, "social networks gives legions of idiots the right to speak when they once only spoke at a bar, after a glass of wine, without harming the community ... but now they have the same right to speak as a Nobel Prize winner. It's the invasion of the idiots" (quoted in Michel 2020).

We react to the government's discourses and to their reiteration or reinterpretation by the media. The chain reaction of behaviors, in connection with communication, is no longer only related to the subject treated, but is the result of the overflow of a mass of information (good and bad) relayed in a viral way by the media and the social networks, and is often the occasion of the upsurge of new viruses.

The phygital offers a new space for socialization through which the apparent autonomy of individuals is constrained by standardized exchanges, but which is also accompanied by a deafening amount of low-quality commentary. A mass of real-time information around the SARS-CoV-2 communication has often lost individuals in *infobesity*, in a *communitagion* of a non-coherent conglomeration of information.

In a phygital world, this unique device should be the object of a real-time analysis of the information, open source and validated by randomly chosen moderators, and made available to users with a broad spectrum decoder, operating, for example, with a system of hyperlinks, a universal guide of good practices or a hotline. Such a system must correspond to the needs of users in health and society (while respecting the diversity of beliefs, i.e. it must not be used as a political or ideological bargain). Similarly, in order to avoid a cognitive overload of all kinds of information, the 1-1-1-1 rule should be recommended: one disease, one site, one treatment and one health.

8.8.2. *Digimal*

After almost two months of total lockdown – from March 17 to May 11, 2020 in France – many people suffered from digital or "digimal" sickness:

> We're getting soft. We can't stand screens anymore. At the beginning of the lockdown, my (only) 9-year-old daughter was Skyping with her friends. Now, she doesn't even want to do that anymore – Laure, 39 (Nicogossian 2020).

The lack of physical encounters and the real-time information flow – of an expanding universe – works against true phygital success, like a cognitive scratch or a scratched vinyl, with the opposite effect of inducing negative emotions in the user. For example, the identification (by password) on multiple sites – necessary for identity protection and cybersecurity – remains non-intuitive and time-consuming, with the disturbing impression of being turned into a dopamine hamster, stuck on frustration–pleasure–reward mechanisms and spending our life pedaling:

> I leave [my 10-year-old daughter] alone to do her homework, she manages on her computer, with the links that the school gives her and her different activities. I'm on a conference call all day, I have a job, I have to keep working. She's fed up, she's not motivated at all – Sophie, 48 (Nicogossian 2020).

8.8.3. *Digital obscurantism*

The desire for improvement and positive management of the health and social crisis has encouraged the deployment of a large number of sites, applications and *connected tools.* A major difficulty, at the user level, concerns the lack of uniformity of the sites and the fact that they are not assembled on a trusted site. We are ultimately under the sway of a multiplicity of digital tools that accelerate the sense of decentering and heteronomy of individuals (Broaweys 2019).

The way the health crisis was handled was by no means perfect, but was it good enough? Some doctors forgot about their patients, some surgeries were postponed and some chronically ill patients did not have access to their treatments. Beyond health, on the educational front, teachers imagined that to ensure "educational continuity" it was enough to send students links and attachments, without worrying about how these documents were received, if at all, on the other side of the screen. A debauchery of sporadically sent attachments made it very difficult for already overworked and family-confined parents to manage their work, their stress and their children. The "pedagogical continuity", as put into practice during the lockdown period was considered a pedagogical aberration by some lucid teachers, well trained in digital tools and aware of the challenge of remote education. Many actors – teachers, students and parents – lacked preparation and were left to their own devices, without any real coordination, and found themselves at odds with the communication link and disconnected from the real needs of "life behind the screen".

Remote communication should not be limited to ensuring that a technology works through the transmission of a message between a sender and a receiver. There is no point in sending information over the Web without considering how the information will be received.

Health technologies adapted to the remote management of patients played the expected role, insofar as 11% of consultations were remote following the announcement of lockdown, compared to less than 1% before this announcement. As for the proportion of doctors who practiced remote consultation, it rose from 11% to 44% between these two periods. However, despite the services provided by remote consultations, some patients suffered from the absence of a physical meeting with their doctor:

> I stay at home. I don't move around anymore. I watch the news on the Internet. But it's terrible, you can't hear a car all day – Claire, 65 (Nicogossian 2020).

> The majority of patients adopted the strategy of mass purchasing in a logic of stocking up before the onset of lockdown, as our study found, with these purchase increases sometimes reaching 20–40%. But as the health situation became critical and fed the fears of chronically ill patients, they sometimes forewent care (ANSM 2020).

Patients with chronic diseases, 20 million in France, lost between the traditional medical system and remote consultation, no longer dared to "bother" their specialists or, for fear of being infected, followed the lockdown to the letter and abandoned all medical follow-ups (Libération, 2020). Conducted during the fifth week of lockdown (mid-April), the EPI-Phare study aimed at analyzing drug consumption habits in relation to Covid-19 noted at this date a return to almost normal consumption of treatments dedicated to chronic pathologies, with a 15 to 30% increase in the delivery of these drugs compared to the beginning of lockdown.

The number of visits to general practitioners in town collapsed at the beginning of the lockdown. Despite the massive implementation of teleconsultations, there was a decrease of around 40% in general medical procedures and 70% in specialty medical procedures:

> We respect the lockdown, we don't go out anymore, because my son has a respiratory problem. We really don't want to catch it! He doesn't even go to see his cousins who live in the house right next door, nothing. He has the Internet. – Paul, 45 (Nicogossian 2020).

Pierre Simon, a leading figure and thinker in telemedicine, questioned the organization of remote monitoring of chronic diseases in the home, highlighting a lack of coordination between city doctors in terms of remote health management in the context of the "Homespital" (Simon 2020). Based on the trend towards digital transformation and redefinition of hospital missions, which had already begun before lockdown, Simon considered it necessary to set up an objective evaluation of the evolution of the French health system and feedback related to lockdown to avoid repeating the dysfunctions that were observed.

8.9. Phygital techniques

"Give thanks to screens and social networks, because they help limit the damage. A gift from heaven for the elderly, talking with their children without being infected, it is a kind of magical improvement of communication transcending physical presence", summarized neuropsychiatrist Boris Cyrulnik. He added, "it's an alteration of the relationship, my computer never smiled at me, never nodded to encourage me or shut me up, etc." (Cyrulnik 2020).

The resources of the digital body are different from those of the physical body. They definitely reduce the physical potentialities; but at the same time, the meeting between the physical body and the digital body is likely to generate new effects that will have to be observed and studied quickly, such as secondary effects, diseases, new knowledge and original therapeutic solutions – and perhaps one day "digital molecules" and "digital therapies".

We can meet on the Internet and invent new physical rituals adapted to the circumstances of a lockdown. Our mental health has become phygital, physical on the one hand, and preciously digital on the other hand. It is necessary in this context to dress up, to get ready, not only to let ourselves become numb, but also to turn on our screen to communicate in a conference call, to adjust the framing of the screen, the blurring of the background and the mute microphone so that the extradiegetic noise does not disturb our interlocutors, all these conditions are soft skills acquired by a good part of France. This technical coordination between the physical and the digital has allowed us to reduce the risks of neurological, psychological and emotional alterations possibly linked to lockdown, by allowing us to maintain a social activity. However, "when the virus is dead, it will be necessary to set up meetings and parties again very quickly, and to lend ourselves to facial expressions, gestures and micro-expressions, because the computer does not allow these ways of communicating" (Cyrulnik 2020).

8.10. Conclusion

In order to ensure the digital transformation of the hospital and to improve the care of tomorrow's health, we have a responsibility to assess the lessons to be learned from lockdown and the imperfections it has brought to light. We must prioritize the development of a health democracy that is supported by the digital transformation.

Lockdown and crisis communication have pushed us to a radicalized use of Internet resources, not only in the field of health and education, but also in that of encounters and sexuality. Not considering the founding practices of our cultural and societal humanity, with the imposed scenario of physical distancing and remote control by the Internet and its tools, leads to the fear of a phenomenon of "the Internet". This brutal deculturation will generate a plastic atrophy of our functions, the paradoxical opposite of a policy of "care taking".

The recent decisions on traceability in times of health crisis, in order to retrieve data from our smartphones for health tracing (INRIA 2020), are questionable in terms of freedoms (France culture 2020) and worry the *Commission nationale de l'informatique et des libertés* (CNIL, French National Commission for Computing and Freedoms)). Lockdown led to a "sudden transformation of the digital health system", which had already begun, accompanied by citizen consultations, but which required more than ever reflection on the ethical principle of "human guarantees" (Gruson 2020). These decisions are notably at the root of questions regarding data sovereignty, as the creation of the health data hub, a platform for hosting all health data, provides for the use of an American host (Vitard 2020).

Communication media are saturated; short, practical and rational information should be gathered, well argued (and fast), accompanied by a guide of good practices and the learning of useful techniques for the phygital body of the lockdown period and that of the post-lockdown period.

Like medicine, the Internet and the digital world are a matter of dose, of prescription, of context. They are both a remedy and a poison, a valuable protection and a misused one, if we systematize their uses without keeping the human being in the loop, if we detach ourselves from the physical world, or if we do not follow the necessary recommendations for digital hygiene, in order to avoid other "viruses".

Encouraging the action of healthy people, carers and volunteers makes it possible to retain meaning and to support the principle of solidarity, without isolating people. Why not use the resources of the Internet and why not create a digital tool – based on the principles of carpooling and geo-localized meetings – in order to solicit, and quickly train, caregivers to contribute to care situations (e.g. by *going to see their neighbors* instead of being afraid of them) and allow them to function? We all need action, affection, physical human presence, social connection and sunshine in the hours we have left.

How can we improve the "failures" of this rich experimentation and activate the key to good health between the contributions of remote technologies and physical communication, a cross between screen and human? This *hybridization of* the living and the digital requires technical and human coordination, so that these technologies work for the good of humanity.

8.11. References

Afnor (2020). Document de référence pour fabriquer des masques barrières [Online]. Available at: https://normalisation.afnor.org/actualites/covid-19-un-document-de-reference-pour-fabriquer-des-masques-barrieres/ [Accessed 08 June 2020].

ANSM (2020). Usage des médicaments en ville Durant l'épidémie… [Online]. Available at: https://www.ansm.sante.fr/S-informer/Points-d-information-Points-d-information/Usage-des-medicaments-en-ville-durant-l-epidemie-de-Covid-19-point-de-situation-apres-cinq-semaines-de-confinement-Point-d-information [Accessed 08 June 2020].

Boumrar, J. and Bordes, M. (2015). Le rôle du facteur humain en gestion des crises. *Communication Sensible* [Online]. Available at: http://www.communication-sensible.com/articles/article296.php [Accessed 08 June 2020].

Broaweys, C. (2019). *La matérialité à l'ère digitale*. PUG, Paris.

Chartier, C. (2020). On ne peut pas sacrifier les jeunes et les actifs pour sauver les vieux. *L'Express* [Online]. Available at: https://www.pressreader.com/france/l-express-france/20200430/282183653205752 [Accessed 08 June 2020].

Citton, Y. (2010). *Mythocratie: Storytelling et imaginaire de gauche*. Éditions Amsterdam, Paris.

Cyrulnik, B. (2020). Boris Cyrulnik: On est dans la résistance, pas encore dans la résilience. *France Culture* [Online]. Available at: https://www.franceculture.fr/emissions/confinement-votre/boris-cyrulnik-on-est-dans-la-resistance-pas-encore-dans-la-resilience [Accessed 08 June 2020].

Dejours, C. (2014). *Le facteur humain*. Presses universitaires de France, Paris.

Dobry, M. (1986). *Sociologie des crises politiques*. Presses de la FNSP, Paris.

Elsevier (2020). Elsevier Covid-19 healthcare hub [Online]. Available at: https://covid-19.elsevier.health/#toolkits [Accessed 08 June 2020].

Faure, O. (2020). Non la France ne traverse pas la plus grande crise sanitaire de son histoire. *Le Figaro* [Online]. Available at: https://www.lefigaro.fr/vox/histoire/non-la-france-ne-traverse-pas-la-plus-grande-crise-sanitaire-de-son-histoire-20200408?fbclid=IwAR0Z2J2b3qtGZ414DK-ihkiDP7-XmuacYSKS7XboTBY0y2K52abvQVJueal#xtor=AL-201 [Accessed 26 May 2020].

France Inter (2020). Le coup de gueule du philosophe André Comte-Sponville sur l'après-confinement. *France Inter* [Online]. Available at: https://www-franceinter-fr.cdn.ampproject.org/c/s/www.franceinter.fr/amp/idees/le-coup-de-gueule-du-philosophe-andre-comte-sponville-sur-l-apres-confinement [Accessed 26 May 2020].

France Musique (2020). Le Boléro de Ravel par l'Orchestre national de France [Online]. Available at: https://www.youtube.com/watch?v=Sj4pE_bgRQI&feature=youtu.be [Accessed 26 May 2020].

Ganascia, J.-G. (2020a). La France va-t-elle espionner les maladies du coronavirus ? *France Culture* [Online]. Available at: https://www.franceculture.fr/sciences/jean-gabriel-ganascia-la-france-va-t-elle-espionner-les-telephones-des-malades-du-coronavirus [Accessed 08 June 2020].

Ganascia, J.-G. (2020b). L'éthique de la recherche en situation de crise sanitaire. *CNRS* [Online]. Available at: https://lejournal.cnrs.fr/billets/lethique-de-la-recherche-en-situation-de-crise-sanitaire [Accessed 08 June 2020].

Gruson, D. (2020). Ethik-IA. *Manager Santé* [Online]. Available at: https://managersante.com/2020/02/24/pourquoi-fallait-il-renforcer-la-garantie-humaine-de-lia-dans-le-projet-de-loi-bioethique-au-senat-reponses-de-david-gruson-et-judith-meh/ [Accessed 11 June 2020].

Illouz, E. (2006). *Les sentiments du capitalisme*. Le Seuil, Paris.

INRIA (2020). Contact tracing et mieux en comprendre les enjeux [Online]. Available at: https://www.inria.fr/fr/contact-tracing-bruno-sportisse-pdg-dinria-donne-quelques-elements-pour-mieux-comprendre-les-enjeux [Accessed 08 June 2020].

Journal international de médecine (2020). Mourir devient une erreur médicale, une interview du Dr Luc Perino. *Journal international de médecine* [Online]. Available at: https://www.jim.fr/medecin/jimplus/tribune/e-docs/_mourir_devient_une_erreur_medicale_une_interview_du_dr_luc_perino_183060/document_edito.phtml [Accessed 08 June 2020].

Kahn, A. (2020). La ligue contre le cancer et la crise du coronavirus. *Ligue contre le cancer* [Online]. Available at: https://www.liguecancer-cd68.fr/coronavirus [Accessed 08 June 2020].

Klein, E. and Brunfaut, S. (2020). Étienne Klein: Aimer la vérité, oui, mais pas déclarer vraies les idées que nous aimons. *L'écho* [Online]. Available at: https://www.lecho.be/dossiers/coronavirus/aujourd-hui-circulent-dans-les-memes-canaux-de-communication-des-connaissances-croyances-informations-commentaires-opinions-et-bobards/10224214.html [Accessed 08 June 2020].

Le Monde (2020). Facebook va avertir les utilisateurs... [Online]. Available at: https://www.lemonde.fr/pixels/article/2020/04/16/facebook-va-avertir-les-utilisateurs-qui-ont-reagi-a-des-messages-dangereux-lies-au-covid-19_6036820_4408996.html [Accessed 08 June 2020].

Lévi-Strauss, C. (1962). *La pensée sauvage*. Plon, Paris.

Lévi-Strauss, C. (1973). *Anthropologie structurale: Deux*. Plon, Paris.

Lévi-Strauss, C. (2004). Lettre de Claude Lévi-Strauss à Wiktor Stoczkowski du 22 novembre. *Cairn* [Online]. Available at: https://www.cairn.info/revue-etudes-2010-4-page-485.htm#no27.

Libération (2020). Deux fois moins d'infractus ce n'est pas normal. *Libération* [Online]. Available at: https://www.liberation.fr/france/2020/04/05/deux-fois-moins-d-infarctus-ce-n-est-pas-normal_1784267 [Accessed 08 June 2020].

Magakian, J. (2006). La créativité à la croisée de trois démarches: Fonctionnalisme, enactment, poétique. *Revue française de gestion*, 161(2), 155–167.

Martin-Juchat, F. (2020). Maintenir la distance: Tristesse à venir d'une socialité sans contact ? *The Conversation* [Online]. Available at: https://theconversation.com/maintenir-la-distance-tristesse-a-venir-dune-socialite-sans-contacts-135736?fbclid=IwAR1aL9xVwX9ETgZkc-sd43Dxbow150wtB_K51odYPAcG6w3sfTGCtKQ3SkI [Accessed 08 June 2020].

Mehrabian, A. and Ferris, S.R. (1967). Inference of attitudes from nonverbal communication in two channels. *Journal of Consulting Psychology*, 31(3), 248–252.

Michel, J.D. (2020). Hydroxychlorine le bal des ignorés [Online]. Available at: http://jdmichel.blog.tdg.ch/archive/2020/04/03/hydroxychloroquine-le-bal-des-ignares-305545.html [Accessed 08 June 2020].

MIT (2014). The importance of feeling. *Technology Review* [Online]. Available at: https://www.technologyreview.com/2014/06/17/172310/the-importance-of-feelings/ [Accessed 08 June 2020].

New York Times (2020). Three cheers for social distancing [Online]. Available at: https://www.nytimes.com/2020/03/27/style/thank-you-for-coming-italy-video-coronavirus.html [Accessed 08 June 2020].

Nicogossian, J. (2020). Étude ethnographique basé sur le vécu des personnes en confinement (qualitative exploratoire).

Noël, X. (2020). Protéger la santé mentale des soignants pour endiguer la pandémie. *The Conversation* [Online]. Available at: https://theconversation.com/proteger-la-sante-mentale-des-soignants-pour-endiguer-la-pandemie-135775 [Accessed 08 June 2020].

Roosevelt, F. (1933). Presidential first inaugural address [Online]. Available at: https://avalon.law.yale.edu/20th_century/froos1.asp [Accessed 08 June 2020].

Routasalo, P. (1999). Physical touch in nursing studies: A literature review. *Journal of Advanced Nursing*, 30, 843–850.

Sanofi Lab Santé (2020). Comment la crise du coronaviorus booste la teleconsultation médicale. [Online]. Available at: https://www.sanofi.fr/labsante/comment-la-crise-du-coronavirus-booste-la-teleconsultation-medicale [Accessed 08 June 2020].

Simon, P. (2020). La télésurveillance médicale des patients atteints de maladies chroniques: Un avant et après Covid-19 ? [Online]. Available at: http://www.telemedaction.org/445654517 [Accessed 08 June 2020].

Tomova, L., Wang, K., Thompson, T., Matthews, G., Takahashi, A., Tye, K., Saxe, R. (2020). The need to connect: Acute social isolation causes neural craving responses similar to hunger. *Biorxiv* [Online]. Available at: https://www.biorxiv.org/content/10.1101/2020.03.25.006643v2 [Accessed 08 June 2020].

Vasak, S. (2020). Y a-t-il un modèle allemand dans la lutte contre le coronavirus ? *France Culture* [Online]. Available at: https://www.franceculture.fr/politique/y-a-t-il-un-modele-allemand-dans-la-lutte-contre-le-coronavirus [Accessed 08 June 2020].

Verweij, M., Senior, T.J., Domínguez, D.J.F., Turner, R. (2015). Emotion, rationality, and decision-making: How to link affective and social neuroscience with social theory. *Frontiers in Neuroscience*, 9, 332.

Vinit, F. and St Pierre, C. (2006). Le toucher dans les soins infirmiers regard croisé entre la discipline infirmière et l'anthropologie. University of Quebec [Online]. Available at: https://docplayer.fr/1415377-Cahier-8-le-toucher-dans-les-soins-infirmiers-regard-croise-entre-la-discipline-infirmiere-et-l-anthropologie.html [Accessed 08 June 2020].

Vitard, A. (2020). Que reproche-t-on au Health Data Hub, attaqué devant le Conseil d'État ? *Usine Digitale* [Online]. Available at: https://www.usine-digitale.fr/article/que-reproche-t-on-au-health-data-hub-attaque-devant-le-conseil-d-etat.N973541 [Accessed 11 June 2020].

Warner, Z. (2020). 1001 Nights of the Wuhan Flue CONFINEMENT Night N°9 "Cracking up" sub English [Online]. Available at: https://youtu.be/ce_hCtkGzgo [Accessed 08 June 2020].

Weick, K.E. (1988). Enacted sensemaking in crisis situations. *Journal of Management Studies*, 25, 305–17.

WFP (2019). Hunger map [Online]. Available at: https://www.wfp.org/publications/2019-hunger-map [Accessed 08 June 2020].

WHO (2019). Drinking water [Online]. Available at: https://www.who.int/en/news-room/fact-sheets/detail/drinking-water [Accessed 08 June 2020].

WHO (2020). Draft landscape of Covid-19 vaccines [Online]. Available at: https://www.who.int/publications/m/item/draft-landscape-of-covid-19-candidate-vaccines [Accessed 08 June 2020].

Worldometers (2020). Covid-19 coronavirus pandemic [Online]. Available at: https://www.worldometers.info/coronavirus/ [Accessed 08 June 2020].

9

Will the Covid-19 Pandemic be an Opportunity to Implement the Principle of Sustainable Development?

9.1. Introduction

An aggressive pandemic is shaking up the certainties of a globalized world and already voices are being raised to announce major changes for the future.

At first sight, it is legitimate to wonder about the excessiveness and dramatization of the effects, as described by information representatives, attributed to this viral attack in the face of a number of victims that is not at all comparable (50 to 100 times lower?) to that linked to the Spanish flu of 1918. High levels of media coverage, greater sensitivity of populations to health risks, fear in front of a difficult to control propagation? There are undoubtedly many reasons for this state of affairs; however, it is not the purpose of this chapter to analyze them.

In just under two months, a key indicator of the global economy, the price of a barrel of oil, plummeted to a negative value and the economic machine seized up.

For many observers, this crisis would be an opportunity to change the rules of the societal game at the global level.

Chapter written by Jean-Paul BOIS-MARGNAC.

What kind of changes might be associated with Covid-19 and its consequences? What are the chances that these changes will become structural at the global level?

First, however, what world are we talking about?

9.2. Economic liberalism: a now dominant ideology

In 1992, after the fall of the Berlin Wall, Francis Fukuyama prophesied the "end of history", meaning the definitive elimination, for the benefit of the market alone, of the ideology advocating state control over the economy and the concomitant socialization of a certain number of "commons".

In the early 1990s, it was difficult to imagine that the triumph of liberalism over communism would undermine the foundations of a political system based on the rule of law and protection of the weak. Some still believed in the utopia of an economy self-regulated by the benefits of the "invisible hand of the market". In fact, this hand led, *a contrario*, to the development of super-monopolies, such as Big Tech (Google, Apple, Facebook, Amazon, Microsoft and others), and while the phenomenon of trusts is not new to the United States, the development of giants of industry, commerce and communication has never had as much impact as it does now on the daily life of the world's population[1].

We now know that the application of the "laissez-faire" doctrine has led to the globalization and financialization of the economy, a system that is difficult for nation-states to control.

Moreover, simply because of the disqualification of their main ideological opponent, communism, the liberal theses underlying world affairs have acquired, in effect, the status of dominant ideology. The concept of dominant ideology, coined by Marxist and Marxian sociologists as part of a global theory of reification/alienation, applies to the present situation in that it never displays itself as dominant, while deeply permeating the perception and behavior of individuals.

Over the decades, there has been a shift from the simple "fetishization of the commodity" (*Les Choses*, Georges Perec, 1965) to the reification/

1 Every month, Facebook has 2.5 billion active users, which are as many economically (and politically) exploitable "profiles".

alienation of the individual consumer, illustrated by the famous advertising slogan: “Because I’m worth it!” If, during the *Trente Glorieuses* (1946–1975, a prosperous period of 30 years in France following the end of the Second World War), some people found virtues in free trade and mass consumption, in the 2000s, tolerable liberalism turned into intolerable ultra-liberalism[2].

Thus, how many citizens, consciously or unconsciously, integrate, through their thirst for consumption, the injunctions of ultra-liberalism? As for the detestable[3] social Darwinism, according to which it is the most apt to survive that survives, this conception of the human adventure is shared by a part of the social body.

Although several movements opposing the effects of unbridled economic liberalism have emerged over the last 20 years, such as Podemos in Spain in 2011 and the *Gilets jaunes* in France in 2018, the influence of these movements has rarely gone beyond the limits of their countries. Similarly, the Occupy movement, launched in 2011 by a group of Canadian activists, which experienced, thanks to the use of social networks, an international audience (London, New York, Montreal and Paris), did not succeed in destabilizing the system.

Endowed with a strong resilience, without any credible ideological opposition, the ultra-liberal ideology thus develops without any real opposition and is even reinforced by serious academic guarantees, which should be examined carefully.

9.3. An effective pragmatics encouraged by argued academic theses

The pragmatics of laissez-faire economics and social Darwinism[4] are based on two mechanisms:

2 Ultra-liberalism is the liberal doctrine taken to its extreme (see below on anarcho-capitalism and libertarianism).

3 It is indeed detestable because this movement has provided the bedrock for State eugenics (United States, Japan, Switzerland, Denmark and Sweden) and its worst deviance, the racist theories of Nazism.

4 The idea of the natural selection of individuals is all the more accepted among Anglo-Saxon Protestants as they recognize the role of “divine anointing” for those who succeed.

– the individuation of consumers/citizens;

– the incentive for the decline of the state.

These pragmatics draw their theoretical foundations – and roadmap – from the theses of anarcho-capitalism and libertarianism[5]. By reading Robert Nozick[6] and Murray Rothbard[7], its theorists, we can see where the completion of the ultra-liberal project could lead. Thus, among the theses developed by these academics, followers of the Vienna School of economics (Ludwig von Mises, Friedrich Hayek), we can note that:

– taxes are equated with hard labor. Redistributive social justice (as advocated by John Rawls) is the antithesis of true justice;

– in the anarcho-capitalist society, each individual is sovereign, their property inviolable. It is up to each individual to protect their person and their sovereign territory;

– "As for the poor, they would not necessarily be less well protected in libertarian anarchy. Are inner-city residents always well protected by the tax-costing public police?"

This argument, based on the philosophy of John Locke (1632–1704)[8], highlights the uselessness (and even the harmfulness) of the State and its regalian functions. It should be remembered that the privatization of these functions is already underway in many countries.

However, under the pressure of the economic crisis caused by Covid-19, States are called upon to play an essential role as economic and social shock absorbers. The underlying question is therefore: should there be more or less State?

---

5 See the essay "L'anarcho-capitalisme et le libertarianisme, feuille de route de l'ultra libéralisme?". Available at: https://www.calameo.com/books/0000173499fc40f64fa93.

6 See the bibliography provided by the Wikiliberal portal: https://www.wikiberal.org/wiki/Robert_Nozick.

7 An extensive bibliography is available at: https://www.wikiberal.org/wiki/Murray_Rothbard_(Bibliographie).

8 For Locke, individuals have an unrestricted right to "life, liberty and property".

9.4. A deceptive "decline"

Thus, in France, under the pressure of successive waves of privatization, the nature of the State as it has been known for 200 years has profoundly changed. It has progressively abandoned its role as producer for that of last resort lender. To assess its disengagement from the country's economy, we need only compare its current influence with the nationalization of entire economic sectors after the Liberation. In contrast, many sectors, such as banking and insurance, expect it to act as a guarantor in the event of default.

This insurance function, which all OECD countries are now playing to the full to cushion the social and economic effects of the crisis, gives credibility to the old slogan: privatize the profits, socialize the losses!

It is therefore the State, in its traditional sense, that protects the weak against the insatiable predation of the strong.

9.5. Suffering from the predations of the deregulated economic order

Those who suffer from deregulation are, first, nature, in the broadest sense of the term (biodiversity, climate change), and second, the most vulnerable populations or social classes. The ideals of the "commons" and the public good have been replaced by a logic of unrestrained monopolization of resources for the benefit of a few: deforestation of primary forests, capture of water resources and rare metals, privatization of life, overfishing and so on.

To an extent that was difficult to imagine in the early 1990s, a globalization without safeguards, without regulation and without a driver has indecently enriched a small class of "persons of independent means", while massively impoverishing the underprivileged classes of the industrialized countries.

However, apart from the subprime crisis, the effects of globalization have only been felt gradually and the resilience of the victims has been such that politicians have been able to content themselves with supporting measures, without having to call into question the principles of the ultra-liberal economy. However, while the repeated warnings of scientists have failed to change the course of our industrial societies towards ecological disaster, the brutality of climate change will force a change in current trajectories with no possible way out.

Once the failure of the insatiable predatory system has been noted, what principles would be able to correct its effects?

9.6. How the post-Covid-19 era could bring about change

In a relationship of both interdependence and rivalry, three superpowers dictate their laws to the entire planet: the United States, China and Europe. Multilateralism, established in 1946 under the aegis of the United States to peacefully settle conflicts between states, is no longer able to counter their selfish and short-termist maneuvers.

Rejected by President Trump's administration, but supported by BRICS (Brazil, Russia, India, China and South Africa), among which China has taken the lead, multilateralism has also shown its limits in the management of the Covid-19 crisis. In April 2020, the last meeting of its highest body, the UN Security Council, was held by video conference and ended in failure.

The same was true in previous decades of specialized forums, such as Earth Summits or Conferences of Parties (COPs), which proved incapable of driving major change.

Therefore, from where could a force emerge that is capable of imposing the necessary change?

Everyone has been able to measure the media impact of a young Swedish woman, Greta Thunberg, both on public opinion and world bodies (COP24, the UN, European Parliament, the Davos Forum, etc.). Would this type of action in favor of the climate be capable of strengthening the dialectical movement already at work between the monolithic block of interests of the globalized economy and the myriad of local initiatives in line with the principles of sustainable development?

As we know, in very everyday actions, each citizen-consumer has a lever for changing production and consumption relationships. Many people in the Western world have already taken this step.

The Covid/19 crisis has led to a proliferation of initiatives: deconstruction-reconstruction of the well-established circuits of globalization, relocalization of certain productions, implementation of short circuits and resocialization through exchange networks. All these practices lead, through a virtuous loop, to a re-evaluation of the "benefits" of consumer society and so on.

However, let us not be naive! An eco-responsible attitude requires renunciations. Therefore, who will be able to make these renunciations in our societies addicted to consumption, irresponsible producers of its corollary, waste? These are renunciations that imply, in particular, renouncing the dogma of indefinite growth at sky-high rates!

Are we fully aware that, as China proclaimed at the presentation of its 13th five-year plan in 2016[9], a 7% growth rate represents a doubling of the wealth produced every 10 years? This is a doubling of production and also, in part, an increase in the consumption of non-renewable resources and pollution.

We must also give up our freedom of movement. In recent years, the expansion of mass tourism has shown its harmful effects in many countries. Examples abound: Machu Picchu, the Taj Mahal, and Venice, which is threatening to sink under the weight of armies of tourists[10].

Here again, for some years now, eco-responsible tourism has been practiced by a few travel agencies, but could such a practice become the rule?

9.7. Principles of sustainable development, foundations of a new social contract

Far beyond James Lovelock's amiable "Gaia hypothesis" (1970) (according to which the Earth is a dynamic physiological system maintaining our planet in harmony with life) or the eco-hippie attitudes of certain ecologists, we must consider the theses of sustainable development as

9 See for reference: https://www.capital.fr/entreprises-marches/le-plan-de-la-chine-pour-doubler-son-economie-en-10-ans-1106931.

10 See for reference: https://www.ledevoir.com/monde/europe/568227/venise-une-ville-noyee-par-le-tourisme.

sources of innovative principles from which we can enact a constitution, laws, regulations[11] and so on.

Thus, a new framework for "living together" could emerge from two major principles:

– limiting predation of any kind in order to ensure the reproduction of resources;

– consideration of the effects of current decisions on the well-being of future generations.

How might these principles lead to a rewriting of the social contract binding most states under the rule of law?

Before answering this question, let us take a quick look back: the Enlightenment gave rise to the shape of the citizen and their inalienable rights guaranteed by the State. Liberal ideology, in contrast, has imposed the figure of the consumer.

In a complete ideological reversal, where the Dominican Henri Lacordaire (1836) asserted, "between Law and anarchy, it is the Law that liberates and anarchy that oppresses", ultra-liberalism retorts, "between anarchy and the Law (the State), it is anarchy that liberates and the Law that oppresses".

The principles of sustainable development go beyond the issue of individual freedom, which is already enshrined in our constitutions, because they aim to preserve the resources essential to survival.

Logically, the limitation of predation of any kind requires that binding rules be adopted internationally and that the political authorities of nation-states have sufficient power to enforce them.

As for the second principle, consideration of the effects of current decisions on the well-being of future generations, unless it is made a constitutional principle, it seems more difficult to put into practice as the mode and spirit of law-making are still so rooted in the short term.

---

11 See the essay "Le Développement Durable". Available at: https://www.calameo.com/books/00001734920e82d5c4621.

9.8. Beyond the citizen and the citizen-consumer, a new political figure

In a Europe made up of empires and kingdoms, the French Revolution inaugurated the nation-state, whose political system was the Republic, which guaranteed the rights not of subjects but of citizens. Although France is still a republic, it can be said that, since the fall of the Berlin Wall and the growing influence of ultra-liberalism, without bloody riots or fury, the historical figure of the citizen has gradually been replaced by that of their consumerist double.

Let us ask ourselves the question: what new figure could give birth to a world applying the principles of sustainable development? What universal figure would be able to accommodate the diversity of political systems? Considering the collapse of our generous idea of universal human rights, this seems utopian. Moreover, how many States reject this idea, States that are often theocracies!

However, there are many signs of the emergence of a planetary awareness of the urgency to adopt new rules to save our planet. Whether by choice or by force, they will eventually be imposed under the pressure of the great waves of migration, through which the hungry and the oppressed will increasingly come to call to account those who have oppressed them. It will therefore not be out of altruism – or a sudden flash of insight – that our affluent societies will change their vision of the world, but under the pressure of phenomena that will overtake them, such as pandemics or uncontrollable migrations induced by climate disorders.

However, this change will be all the more accepted and accompanied if it responds to a moral requirement.

9.9. Towards a new morality

The demand for a moral code of conduct in public life seems to be an aspiration that is increasingly shared. Yes, it is indeed morality that we need and those who suffer from its absence in public life are ready, in order to find one, to follow a principle dictated by the *good*.

Beyond the obvious need to fight corruption, an endemic scourge in almost all societies, beyond even a moral code of conduct, a moral code of living better and of preserving the future, inspired by the two principles of sustainable development, appears to be the foundation around which the expectations of the most threatened populations and individuals could be united.

As mentioned above, the proponents of ultra-liberalism, libertarians and anarcho-capitalists, also claim a moral basis, drawn in this case from Lockean philosophy, which would itself be modeled on a natural right, as a direct emanation of a "state of nature".

The postulate of these currents of thought consists of affirming that "what comes from nature is right and good"[12]. Thus, to establish the rules of living together, a human society would only have to draw inspiration from the rules of nature.

Rousseau, in contrast to the previous idea, states that he wants to "substitute a moral and legitimate equality for what nature may have placed of physical inequality between men, [such] that, being unequal in strength or genius, they all become equal by convention and by right" (*The Social Contract*, 1762).

Behind these opposing ideologies lies a double presupposition on the question of the good: who dictates it (nature, the State)? Who is to benefit (class, individual, citizen)? It remains for us to choose.

At the present time, after having experimented with different social systems, all of which have more or less shown their limits, we find ourselves faced with an empty page. We sense that a new balance – around the notion of "the good" – must be found between the State, the citizen, the market, nature and so on, but what kind?

It is a complex equation with *n* solutions. Could we move from a "state of nature" to a "right of nature", where we recognize the rights (without reciprocal duties) of its representatives: animal and plant species, oceans and primary forests?

---

12 Nazi ideology took up the same reasoning, according which the "old German" – or the German of "pure race" – holds the truth; see Johann Chapoutot's *La loi du sang* (Gallimard, 2014).

This is undoubtedly possible, but only if we accept the abandonment of our anthropocentric vision that places us at the summit of creation. The human is a living organism like any other, but because of our domination over nature – acquired over the millennia – we have duties towards it[13]. For several decades now, a philosophical current has been working to reinforce this just attitude, notably involving Tom Regan, Peter Singer, Boris Cyrulnik, Florence Burgat and Elisabeth de Fontenay.

9.10. Conclusion: uncertainty and unpredictability

If repeated droughts, devastating floods and the inevitable rise in water levels are all factors capable of altering the balance of power between lesser nations and superpowers, a pandemic such as Covid-19 also forces the human race, a fragile passenger on a tiny (and unique) spaceship, to examine its conscience.

In our developed countries, the Covid-19 episode is more than a simple paradigm shift, it is rather the equivalent of the tilting of the magnetic poles in the history of the Earth, the prodigious moment when, according to the beautiful formula, those who do the chores replace the first to climb in the collective representation.

This is true during the crisis, but what about afterwards? What are the chances of a profound change in our lifestyles, consumption patterns and social organization? Will this pole shift be permanent or temporary?

Could it be, for example, that the populations constituting Europe will succeed in imposing a new political and economic model and that, by contagion, the underlying principles will have a small chance of spreading throughout the world?

The great complexity of our interdependencies makes any forecasting illusory.

Let us admit that, like any complex system, the post-Covid world is unpredictable.

---

13 The French Parliament recently enshrined in law that animals are "sentient beings" and no longer mere objects.

Everything is growing, everything is potential.

For all the reasons mentioned in this article, will the Covid-19 episode be the spark that sets the prairie on fire?

9.11. References

Bois-Margnac, J.-P. (2012). Le développement durable, fondement d'une nouvelle philosophie politique en réplique aux violences de la globalisation? [Online]. Available at: https://www.calameo.com/read/000017349f435b5e8740e.

Bois-Margnac, J.-P. (2018). About sustainable development [Online]. Available at: https://www.calameo.com/read/0000173492ae6f707cdac.

Bois-Margnac, J.-P. (2019). Anarcho-capitalisme et libertarianisme [Online]. Available at: https://www.calameo.com/read/0000173499fc40f64fa93.

Carré, S. (2009). *La pensée libertarienne*. Presses universitaires de France, Paris.

Fukuyama, F. (2018). *La fin de l'histoire et le dernier homme*. Flamarion, Paris.

Lemieux, P. (1985). *Du libéralisme à l'anarcho-capitalisme*. Presses universitaires de France, Paris.

Lemieux, P. (1988). *L'anarcho-capitalisme*. Presses universitaires de France, Paris

Nozick, R. (1993). *Anarchie, État et utopie*. Presses universitaires de France, Paris.

Rawls, J. (2001). *Justice as Fairness: A Restatement*. Harvard University Press, Cambridge.

10

The Pandemic Has Invited Itself into a World in the Midst of a Crisis of Meaning

10.1. Foreword

The current health crisis has stunned us. It will lead us to an end that no one knows. We hoped the warm days of summer would liberate us, but we are still waiting. Our socio-economic models have been seriously disrupted by Covid-19. We will get back on our feet but, at this moment in time, we do not yet know how and where to turn; this is a path that has been well prepared by singular thought.

At this point, we still do not know what we will be able to imagine, create, implement or how quickly it will all be made possible.

"This virus is a filthy thing", say our most eminent doctors. Therapeutic strategies are still in their infancy. The duration and even the concept of acquired immunity are the subject of uncertain debate: how many successive assaults could we be condemned to endure? The vaccine will take many months to develop, and even longer to be validated by the health authorities. Beyond that, we must now prepare ourselves for other episodes of this type. H1N1, HIV, Ebola and SARS warned us; the threat exists.

Chapter written by Philippe TRONC.

After the health ordeal, we will have to deal with the economic consequences. The lives sacrificed, shortened and abused seem to weigh very little in the end compared to the disorganization of entire sectors of the economy. All of this uncertainty weighs on how we can plan for the future.

At this stage, we have no ambition to play futurologist: this role requires a very broad (too broad for us) overview of the situation on many levels. Furthermore, in a way, this role remains rather thankless because, as Jean Staune says very well, “a good futurologist knows how to say what is sure to happen, but never specifies the timeframe”. Faced with so many difficulties, we are certainly not giving up and we have the ambition to participate in the emergence of the “world after”, if there is one (there will be, but will it be different?). There is an apparent broad consensus that “the after will be different”. The forces of normalization are at work, however, even though there is a magnificent windfall effect, through the current health crisis, for the ecological discourse.

However, we already know what we no longer want and we are trying to express it today. It is not a question of burning witches, thus evacuating all subjects, exonerating ourselves from a collective responsibility in a moment of exaltation and emotion without a future, following the example of what social networks are doing today, which are taking over from the expiatory ceremonies of the Place de Grève (the main Parisian place of executions under the *Ancien Régime*[1] and the Revolution, today the Place de l’Hôtel de Ville).

It is simply a question, and this is already very presumptuous, of ensuring that the crisis we are experiencing never happens again; or, to put it mildly, of doing our best to ensure that such a crisis never happens again. We must now fear that the end of the crisis will be an atmosphere of settling of scores. This may not be desirable but things must be said, which is, in my opinion, one of the conditions for resilience.

Those responsible will have to face their guilt this time. They will also have to learn from their behavior in order not to commit – again – the fatal errors of the present time. We will simply avoid shaving their heads, scorning them or insulting them, thus showing that the experience of the past

1 The political and social system of France from the Late Middle Ages to the French Revolution in 1789.

century has made us grow in our humanity, and that the future must be built with a certain amount of humility.

10.2. Giving meaning

The pandemic has invited itself into a world in the midst of a crisis of meaning.

Last year, I invited a series of speakers to Castres (Tarn, France) related to the theme of "giving meaning" so that together we could all try to distinguish the motivations of a true meaning given back to life, initially through the entrepreneurial projects of the participating company directors. There were, among others, a leading futurologist, an eminent technology expert, an admirable bionic painter, a poet–singer–entertainer, the only human resources director I have ever met, a mathematician who was totally disrupted and block-chained, and an anthropologist lost in the middle of the North Pole. The meeting was lovely and fruitful.

Moreover, the younger generations are calling us to account on the subject of "meaning". The independent researcher Jean Staune talks about this issue with great relevance in his book *Les Clés du futur* (2019). In fact, each person builds up a patchwork of beliefs, which gives a particular and specific meaning to their existence.

The challenge for organizations is to bring about and propose a common meaning. This is a long-term, iterative and agile task, heuristic to a certain extent, and one that comes up against the expression of powers that are all too often short-termist.

The current pandemic has clearly demonstrated our inability to manage this "meaning". The emergency contributed to this incapacity and still contributes to it for many; however, the absence of the beginnings of a shared vision is an even more significant factor in this difficulty.

In this tangle of shattered lives created by the health crisis, how can we reconcile the short-termism born of a countable vision of the efficiency of the healthcare system, which appears to be far removed from the Hippocratic Oath, according to which the doctor irrevocably commits themselves to defending humanity and life?

How can we hear, without impulsively throwing out his words, the French philosopher André Comte-Sponville when he states:

> The vast majority of us will not die from the coronavirus. I was very struck by this sort of collective panic that gripped the media first, but also the public, as if all of a sudden we were discovered to be deadly. This is not really a scoop. We were deadly before the coronavirus, we'll be deadly after.

I would like him to explain his position to my niece, who has separated herself from her only child in order to devote herself to her job as a resuscitator specialized in Covid-19; my niece who cries on her way home for having put a new patient in "prone position" (a last resort that aims to help patients breathe better). However, does André Comte-Sponville, through his words, not express some essential truths that allow us to find meaning and put this chaotic period we are living through into perspective?

Today, power is only subsequent to Médiamétrie polls (a company specializing in media audience measurement). De Gaulle must be turning in his grave. Water has passed under the bridge but this attitude, especially in times of crisis, makes us doubt, due to its opportunism, any vision even at the highest levels. "We must be sure that the captain's hat is pointing towards the port, no matter what tacks he and his boat (in this case, ours) take (in order to cross the finish line)", as Jean Staune says. This is not the case at present, not because of the tacks made by our "frail boat", but because these tacks are suffered and give the impression that the compass has been lost. In fact, the uncertainty has somehow destabilized us.

We want meaning for tomorrow, common to each of the meanings we give individually. We no longer want a short-term approach, with a rhythm that is too clearly electoral, tending towards re-election, which is in a way the politician's "grail". The expression of democracy is no longer guaranteed by a pile of pyramidal organizations that oversee the democratic process. The time has come for sharing, direct expression, confrontation and debate. This is a delicate exercise, but who said that the exercise of power was simple?

10.3. Crisis in personal behavior

In crisis situations, the emphasis is on interpersonal behavior. This involves two main elements: altruism and otherness. Here again, it is clear that we are far from perfection.

As far as altruism is concerned, we have largely delegated our concern for others and the common good. Short moments of remission still pave the way to a more harmonious world, largely supported by communication tools that promote the expression of collective emotion. However, for the most part, we make up for our long eclipses of empathy through the 8 p.m. applause that rises from our windows and balconies, in the direction of the health professionals to whom we have rather cowardly delegated the task of repairing the coronavirus attacks. So, is it a matter of respect and admiration for them and necessary introspection for us?

What about otherness? Are we capable, there too, of taking into account the Other in all their singularity? The exaltation of the period leaves the field open to all kinds of incongruities in this area. Invective, accusations, fake news from self-proclaimed specialists and all kinds of deception show how little respect we have for the Other.

It is time to institute a debate on the ideas, ethical reflection and moral principles necessary for any political orientation back to the fore, and this other than by means of framed, botched, often obfuscated consultations and, moreover, without any restitution other than the vote on articles of law in front of an empty hemicycle. Obsessed with the utilitarian, we refuse to take a step back at the right time, when it would be appropriate to do so, that is, outside times of crisis. We debate at the wrong time, when we should be showing unfailing solidarity in action.

In sport, rugby shows us an example of a community of action carried by values of unfailing support, a community through which disagreements arising from the game are settled in the changing room. In the business world, we do not hesitate to say, for example, that "every great organization has a great board". It is a shame we do not know how to take such a statement into account in our personal and social lives.

10.4. Crisis of business models

In his fascinating essay *Le capitalisme est-il moral?*, Comte-Sponville closes the debate with:

> Capitalism is neither moral nor immoral. It is of another order, of the mechanical order *a priori*. The apple that fell on Newton's nose was neither moral nor immoral. It underwent the mechanical effect of the earth's attraction and crushed the poor boy's nose.

Capitalism is a "bazaar thing", into which we put money in order to get as much as possible (a lot) out of it. The use that we make of it, in contrast, brings us back to ethics and leads us to say, through the law, what is allowed and what is not.

As for the theorists of ultra-liberalism, they continue to celebrate a hype of convergence and infinite regulation. Certain bitter failures of industrial policies sacrificed on the altar of financialization, projects such as the DMP (*dossier medical partagé*, shared medical file) and the delay in e-health, can at least partly be explained by this recurrent desire for self-regulation. Realism forces us to develop a minimum of control mechanisms, even though we keep in mind the myth of the "noble savage" (idealization of humans in the state of nature). We must exercise caution, however, because too much regulation plunges us into the indecision and immobility that we have seen play out too much in the societal crisis that we are currently experiencing.

10.5. Crisis of our social models

Analysis of the behavior of different countries with regard to the Covid-19 pandemic shows how much influence social models can have on our ability to face these new perils.

It is interesting to note that at the time of writing, the majority of the victims of the pandemic are in the highly developed Western nations. These societies are marked by the way they operate as rich and affluent societies with bloated economies. We are no longer used to confronting perils that call into question our short-term ability to survive. We have the insolent certainty that we can no longer be put in fundamental difficulty.

We have time, we can search endlessly for perfection, we fight risk-taking, whereas life itself is a risk and is fundamentally a struggle, even though our honor consists of making people forget it. We try to project ourselves into a sanitized future, we speculate, we leave the earth of reality for the ether and we are no longer able to apprehend the immediate, the essential. We produce entropy by superimposing regulations that may be adapted to our "normal" situation as wealthy people, but that are certainly out of step with the crisis situation we are experiencing.

We have subjected our political decisions to the economy, to the useful, to finance. A CEO is now received like a head of state. Transnational powers have been established, including Big Tech (Google, Apple, Facebook, Amazon, Microsoft and others), that bypass the sovereignty of the people, which is nevertheless necessary for the urgent management of the crisis, especially at the local level.

The writer and philosopher Éric Sadin expresses this idea vehemently when he talks about the hold of an omnipresent techno-liberalism, a progressive societal resignation and submission to a technological *deus ex machina*, telling us what is good and what is bad.

My intention is not to reject everything. In fact, is that possible? However, I do intend to participate in the reactivation of the reflexes (I dare not say "implementation of the processes") that are essential to have in an emergency. A friend of mine who is an emergency doctor used to tell me – and I believe him – that his job was close to that of a horse trader. What does that mean? Simply that when he makes the decision for an EVASAN (aeromedical evacuation), he is not sure of anything in terms of diagnosis. He decides "simply", using the limited data he has, with the feeling he has in connection with the patient's complaint and the clinical picture. He works with a certain degree of intuition. Faced with imminent danger, risk-taking – which goes beyond procedures, good practices, recommendations and so on – is necessary.

This is a far cry from the decision-making system used when conducting double-blind trials for the purpose of testing the advantage of a new therapeutic strategy that is supposed to eliminate the risk. A few dramatic cases in recent years have clearly shown the limits of this assertion, and current discussions on the use of cohorts in real-life data clearly illustrate the difficulties encountered by mathematical modeling, the necessity of which we, of course, do not deny (would we have the legitimacy to do so?).

The point here is to argue for a true cohabitation of the two approaches (classic trials and follow-up of volunteers in real-life conditions), which must, when an emergency context requires it, cohabit in such a way as to respect and complement each other, rather than confront each other.

Human life cannot be reduced to a series of algorithms any more than social relationships or the economy. Models certainly allow us to approach reality; however, they do not enable us to solve it. To take a back seat to technocracy is a kind of refusal of obstacle for politicians. In this respect, we must remember that horses that refuse to jump a hurdle in a competition are not qualified for the next competition!

10.6. The health crisis as seen from France

In January 2020, the message regarding Covid-19 in France was as follows: "The risk of infection from Wuhan is almost zero, the risk of spreading the coronavirus in the population is very low"[2]. In mid-May, 30,000 deaths were recorded in the country. France crossed the threshold of 70,000 deaths on January 16, 2021[3].

Warning signs and alerts from the World Health Organization that were poorly taken into account and haphazard crisis communication progressively discredited by successive lies and by the very difficult to integrate impact of social networks – these were the elements at the basis of the bad management, in France and elsewhere, of the coronavirus crisis. Nevertheless, the bankruptcy of the French healthcare system was avoided thanks to the remarkable dedication of health professionals on the ground, the health strategy that was followed having nevertheless led France to find itself in the top five nations in terms of the number of deaths per million inhabitants. Who would have thought that a healthcare system as renowned as the French one would have achieved such a result?

At the same time, the outlook for the coming months and years is uncertain. How did we arrive at such a conclusion? Overall, and without wishing to return to what has been said above, there are few fundamentally perverse societal systems, but many more foolish ways of making them

2 Agnès Buzyn on exiting the Council of Ministers on January 24, 2020. Replay available on France TV Info.

3 See https://www.francetvinfo.fr/sante/maladie/coronavirus/covid-19-la-france-franchit-le-seuil-des-70-000-morts-avec-1.

work. While a certain number of errors have been corrected since the beginning of the current health crisis, a few still remain and we will have to rectify them.

In this regard, we must consider that managing a health system is first and foremost a matter of balancing the supply of care and patient demand. This leads to a whole series of elements, as listed below.

1) *Linking patient expectations with the supply of care as closely as possible.* Geographic information systems have been mature enough for many years to be used as information and knowledge media. Furthermore, for as many years, geography has been considered a mere attribute, not a structuring dimension. The quality of a healthcare system is driven notably by its accessibility and by its adequacy to the populations in a given territory. The current crisis has highlighted many questions on this point. A consolidated vision of resources is more than difficult when it is not based on a stable reference point, which can only be the territory.

2) *Implementing tools to detect the emergence of phenomena.* These may include geo-epidemiology and segmentation of populations in a healthcare supply basin, such as the *Groupements hospitaliers de territoire* (GHTs) in France. Controlling the Covid-19 pandemic, with the absence of effective preventive or curative therapeutic solutions for the time being, relies largely on detailed knowledge of the distribution of vulnerable populations and epidemic outbreaks.

3) *Implementing analysis tools.* Despite what some may say, life is multifactorial. We must therefore have the tools to study the statistical links between health and the environment in the general sense of the term. Of course, in this sense, we need to have access to big data, which is at the service of the art of finding what we are not looking for. However, again, we need to consider the geographical visualization of data in a precise manner. To illustrate our thinking in the field of oncology, for example, it is necessary to drastically develop our cancer registers in France, which have remained at a shockingly underdeveloped stage despite the good will of doctors, often retired, who are trying to give them meaning and content[4].

4) *Establishing steering tools.* In the context of the Covid-19 crisis, it took weeks to see the appearance of a few content sites that were nevertheless largely inadequate, especially when they were under the control

4 For more information, see https://www.hsph.harvard.edu/gis/links/.

of the authorities. Completely out of step with the current practices of the population, their responsiveness appeared weak and their readability unsatisfactory, despite some isolated successes. Private initiatives, such as "Covid-minute", slowed down however by means that are difficult to mobilize, have done better.

5) *Setting up logistical tools.* All of the episodes of the crisis that have already occurred highlight the logistical difficulties of being "close" to the patient. Various supplies show a significant gap between the needs and the means put in place to meet them, for example delays in obtaining test results.

6) *Mobilizing health professionals.* This should go without saying, but how? None of my friends who work in the city had a precise idea of their potential involvement in the implementation of "white plans" (organization protocols planned in advance by the health authorities to deal with exceptional health situations). No simulation had been undertaken ex ante for this type of mobilization. In the industry, fire simulations are commonplace. Is this again a matter of money? In order to implement white plans, training and information materials, coordination tools and exchange blogs are essential elements that should be made available to all healthcare structures. Some doctors in the Albi region have come together, on their own initiative, around digital communication and collaboration tools to give meaning to their fight against Covid-19.

7) *Testing patients for SARS-CoV-2.* This should go without saying, but where? Home testing is probably the safest. What if we relied on the network of 25,000 proximity points made up of pharmaceutical pharmacies to do this? These pharmacies are having difficulty finding their place in the health system's value chain, even though they are supported by an information system that is already operational (the implementation of the pharmaceutical file at the expense of the DMP at the time was quite significant). We like to dream of a world in which pharmacists, who are truly competent professionals, would be given their rightful place, in a context in which community medicine and hospitals would be de-siloed, and in which collaboration between health professionals would progress beyond parochial disputes. Here too, training and information, blogs and coordination and management of the resources needed to provide the service are essential elements that should be made available.

8) *Making the relationship between ambulatory medicine and the hospital more fluid.* The coronavirus crisis has once again shown the inadequacy of communication between ambulatory and hospital medicine

and the hospital. Many doctors have put their private practice activities on hold to make themselves available to hospital services. However, in the end, very few were integrated into the battle plan. Unpreparedness, white plans never tested. Operational emergencies cannot be improvised. They are prepared, rehearsed and learned. The shared medical file, which has been poorly attended since 2004, is proving to be a major and necessary element in the current health crisis. The DMP is, in fact, both a vehicle for information and coordination and a medium for a medical service (teleconsultation), as well as a potential basic tool for artificial intelligence (AI) applied to health. For its implementation, the suspicion still present regarding the use of the data remains to be settled. The Orwellian specter still looms large. This DMP is the cornerstone of a genuine rollout of telehealth. However, the current crisis has had an extremely virtuous effect on the deployment of digital tools that increase the capabilities of healthcare professionals: during the Covid-19 pandemic, Digilence and Medvir[5] (medical intelligence services) implemented an AI tool allowing everyone to take stock of their health situation. The principles of these services are based on empowering the patient with respect to their own health and diagnostic assistance for the general practitioner, relieving congestion in the emergency services and monitoring the health sequence. The post-Covid period must be devoted to consolidating these first significant deployments in the structure recommended in *Ma santé 2022* (a collective commitment to health proposed by the French government as a global response to the health challenges facing France), as well as to extending the services made available to patients and professionals. As with any tool, it is not enough, and within the framework of *Ma santé 2022*, the health territories, embodied in the GHTs, must be governed by patients and hospital staff, and also by professionals working in the field of community medicine. In this respect, the French Hospital Federation (*Fédération hospitalière de France*, FHF), which groups together French medico-social and public health establishments, is introducing an approach known as "population responsibility", which is based on a new fluidity – to be consolidated – between ambulatory medicine and the hospital. It is an approach centered on a segmented population, with a view to the overall care of the person throughout their life by means of protocols decided in advance[6].

---

5 For more information, see https://medvir.fr.

6 For more information, see https://www.reseau-hopital-ght.fr/actualites/l-approche-populational-or-the-cultural-revolution-in-health.html.

9) *Debunking the medical and social services.* Is it possible to do nothing about one of the most terrible scandals of the Covid-19 epidemic? Elderly people died en masse in the EHPADs (*Établissements d'hébergement pour personnes âgées dépendantes*, accommodation for dependent elderly people) in France, sometimes without us doing our "best" to save them. In this regard, I can hear Comte-Sponville's speech[7], quoted above, which can be summarized as follows: "Why do you stay with the dead and the old? Take care of the living instead." Nevertheless, we can question the values of a society that does not sufficiently protect its elderly, justifying negligence through technical and economic choices. The *Cour des comptes* (French financial jurisdiction in charge of controlling the regularity of public accounts), in a 2005 report that was too quickly buried[8], recommended breaking down the barriers, particularly at the economic level, by highlighting the fact that we did not have the means to take care of our elderly other than through a strong intergenerational solidarity approach. In the end, nothing or almost nothing has been done in 20 years, and the EHPADs are still operating without a doctor available at night within a reasonable time, and with too few staff compared to their numbers of residents – around 80 on average. It is therefore time to integrate all that telemedicine can bring to the life of the Ehpad and increase the number of employees in direct contact with our elderly.

10) *Implementing healthcare pathways.* One of the lessons of the pandemic is the doubt that has been cast on the level of excellence of the French health system. France is both the fifth largest economy in the world and one of the top five nations with the highest rates of deaths attributable to Covid-19. Even though we can argue about absolute measurements, the ratios of people affected by the epidemic are higher than we would have expected in view of certain nearby countries and the resources that we devote to health (even though questions remain about their allocation). The French health system continues to suffer from a certain lack of efficiency. In the end, it is more a care system than a health system. Nosocomial diseases, health problems of iatrogenic origin and duplications of procedures are the major dysfunctions that the French health system must try to improve, in

7 For more information, see https://www.franceinter.fr/idees/le-coup-de-gueule-du-philosophe-andre-comte-sponville-sur-l-apres-confinement.

8 Cour des comptes. Les personnes âgées dépendantes: Rapport au Président de la République suivi des réponses des administrations et des organismes intéressés. Available at: https://www.vie-publique.fr/rapport/27719-les-personnes-agees-dependantes-rapport-au-president-de-la-republique.

particular by implementing the concept of "healthcare pathways". The shift from a "heroic and curative" health system to one that is more heavily oriented towards prevention, or even prediction, which is now possible, is a major axis of progress in health efficiency. This is because, as we know from industry, quality approaches must be implemented as soon as possible to avoid costs and to take better account of people. All of this only exists in the inclusive perspective that is the health pathway. Hervé Pingaud and Elyes Lamines at Isis in Castres (an engineering school specializing in e-health) have been working on this subject at the university level. The will to take this direction seems to be emerging from all the stakeholders. Putting health actions into perspective, based on the capitalization of knowledge, is a prerequisite for the implementation of new economic and remuneration models for healthcare workers that are likely to replace the current models, which have been so decried, but which have nonetheless made it possible to structure the notion of "activity" within healthcare institutions.

Making a health system work also means counting on reliable and shared data. We have been discussing the interoperability of health IT systems since 2004. The DMP, which was launched at that time, was a matter for IT specialists, and the trench warfare that took place at the time has lasted. We need a standard, but mostly my standard, we heard. We are gradually emerging from this cacophony under the guidance of numerous committees and agencies. Later, there was talk of syntactic interoperability. In standardized pipes, we would exchange messages that were also standardized. Now we come to "semantic interoperability": last but not least! In messages with defined formats conveyed in standardized "pipes", the same terms would be used to say the same things. Behind repositories, dictionaries and lexicons, such as the *Systematized Nomenclature of Medicine – Clinical Terms* (SNOMED CT) or the International Classification of Diseases (ICD), there remains usage. This is where the problem lies!

It seems to us that we should implement back-office approaches to ensure unification on the basis of the exact terms used by each person, rather than imagining that health professionals, who are angrily independent, should be forced to follow a pre-established code. Accepted convergence is a cultural matter and therefore a matter of generations. We do not have the time.

Quality data are rarely native. They have to be acquired. Data never constitute knowledge but require patient and organized consolidation to become it. This raises the question of monetization. We advocate an approach that is as civic-minded as possible: a voluntary and ethical approach, like donating blood or platelets. "Give your data" as you do for your blood, and thus contribute to saving lives. Remuneration for the work undertaken to make the data usable is necessary, but the data itself must be free.

Making a health system work is thus learning to work together. The "circus" maintained by the media and by ourselves through social networks is the expression of the parochial quarrels that largely occupy our health system. The quarrels of specialists, methodological declarations in moments that required coherence and action, continue to ruin the confidence that users may have in it. The crisis has made them apparent to all. Decision-making processes are generally not designed to extract themselves from even the most common cognitive biases. The structures that govern our healthcare system are largely populated by individuals who are certainly very respectable, but all trained in the same mold, following the same paths. How can we escape the confirmation bias, for example, that will lead them to seek solutions adapted to their common analyses and cultures? Exiting a crisis often requires thinking "outside the box". The gap between decision-makers and field workers has proved to be abysmal. The situation was saved by the grassroots movements, almost in spite of the leaders. The time has come for diversity and collaboration in ecosystems. They bring richness and relevance. Digital technology is at the service of this diversity and collaboration.

Making a health system work means providing the right resources at the right time. At the right time means being prepared and managing the emergency. This is a real job, and crisis management cannot be assumed by those who manage business as usual. The current crisis has been a recurring reminder of this since it began. On the subject of the "right resources", we have found that globalization is an obstacle to our survival after it was hailed as necessary or favorable to liberal capitalism. We will not go into the many twists and turns of masks, respirators, anesthesia products, tests, candidate molecules for vaccines and treatments and so on. We have relocated products that have proved to be strategic for reasons essentially of profitability, relocating profits to low-tax areas. We still have to take the return ticket, because in reality, the crisis is managed on the ground, in proximity, *hic et nunc* (Biot 2020).

Making the health system work also means helping it to be innovative. The Covid-19 crisis was a caricature of expert disputes. Yet these disputes were not appropriate when it came to saving lives. The "intergalactic" clinical trials failed to provide answers in the necessary time frame. Conventional decision-making and development processes for new therapeutic strategies proved inadequate. Progress has been made and "performance" achieved, but not to the level required. All quality processes involve what were called "degraded processes" in the old days and are now called "bypass processes". It is time to ask the question: how can we drastically increase our agility?

The development of therapeutic molecules seems to be very difficult to achieve in the French model. In this respect, the *Health Data Hub*[9], recommended by the health authorities to facilitate the sharing of data from a wide variety of sources in order to promote research, is an initiative that should be accelerated. However, it is also urgent to provide the keys to the widest possible use of this initiative, while promoting the rights of individuals to their sensitive data. Should the implementation of shared information processing tools not also be studied, so that innovative start-ups can devote themselves to the clinical proof of concept, rather than to the implementation of excessively expensive infrastructures? Would this approach not also put a stop to cost inflation?

The conspiracy debates of recent times have, as always, the interest of highlighting certain flaws. The supposed (or real) interests of pharmaceutical companies have been used, fueled by shocking statements by certain executives. So what solutions should we find and implement so that the race to the double-digit net profit of pharmaceutical companies stops? What actions should be taken, for example regarding intellectual protection in order to take into account the short period of return on investment, which sometimes generates aberrant price demands and the establishment of costly technical barriers to entry (extreme purification of active ingredients and many other galenic works that do not necessarily have any therapeutic value). Furthermore, what limits should be placed on the protection policies that demand ever more clinical cases, without improving the statistical quality of the results? What solutions can be found in order to leave room for research on rare diseases, where the "market" is so small that the unfortunate patients suffering from these diseases are left to their fate, as they are not "profitable"?

9 For more information, see https://www.health-data-hub.fr.

We need not only an innovative system, of course, but also a secure one, because there is no such thing as zero risk or zero defects. Excellence cannot be a management tool, but the requirement is certainly the foundation. In this context, we must finally recognize that the arsenal – very finely honed – of classic clinical studies is not likely to represent the real exploitation of the molecule or device. Drug evaluation studies must be extended on the basis of cohorts and real-life data. Perhaps then we will be able to avoid events like the recent and odious scandals (on this subject, see the dissertation on evidence-based medicine by Jacques Massol (2016)).

10.7. Conclusion

Like all major crises, the Covid-19 pandemic provides us with many lessons. We have tried to describe what we no longer want and what we see as the way forward. We hope to learn from this and implement actions that will allow us to respond effectively to the next virus, move forward in our values and express our generosity and empathy.

The crisis has shown that healthcare workers in the field are both heroic and generous. It is a burning obligation for civil society to revisit its expectations of a demanding and methodical health system.

Let us put the issues in the right places: ethics and morality are at the source. The law indicates what is allowed and what is not, within the "possibilities" defined above.

The rest is a question of implementation, which does not mean that it is simple. On the contrary, let us refuse to take erratic steps and, together, let us validate that "the captain's hat is pointing towards the port, no matter what tacks he takes".

10.8. References

Biot, J. (2020). Mission stratégique visant à réduire les pénuries de médicaments essentiels: Rapport au Premier ministre. 18 June [Online]. Available at: https://www.vie-publique.fr/rapport/274702-mission-strategique-pour-reduire-les-penuries-de-medicaments-essentiels.

Lamine, E. (2019). Sur la transformation numérique des organisations, en particulier dans le domaine de la Santé. ISIS/HDR/INP, Toulouse.

Massol, J. (2016). L'"Evidence Based Medicine" (EBM): Utile reflet de la réalité ou dangereux miroir de sorcière ? Master's thesis, University of Paris 1 Panthéon-Sorbonne, Paris [Online]. Available at: https://dumas.ccsd.cnrs.fr/dumas-01431212/document.

Sadin, E. (2020). *L'ère de l'individu tyran, la fin d'un monde commun*. Grasset, Paris.

Staune, J. (2019). *Les clés du futur: Clé du monde demain*. Les Éditions de l'Observatoire, Paris.

Conclusion

When Philippe Simon and I began thinking about this book, the idea was that of a "post-world" emerging after the end of a first world cut in two (the West vs. the rest of humanity), with a dichotomy regulated by institutions, and through a second world structured by asymmetrical warfare between powers and terrorism. Due to illness, Philippe Simon left his place to Jacques Barnouin, who was able to complete this work with me. These two divisions of the world that have just been mentioned still exist and are still the subject of crises, as evidenced by the attacks that regularly shake the planet and have just impacted France.

The Covid-19 crisis is adding crisis to crisis. Covid-19 is an emerging disease for which appropriate responses must be provided. However, it is not just any emerging disease, because the epidemic spread by the SARS-CoV-2 coronavirus is following in the footsteps of globalization. It is a clear sign of this, an unavoidable consequence. For the pandemic has spread through the explosion of air transport, the global society and the frenzy of exchanges, imitations and generalizations, as well as the crossroads of uses, goods, people, life paths and viruses. Before finding serenity, we will have to face the viruses of others, and they will have to face our multi-resistant bacteria. We will have to exchange our pathogens and little by little affirm our defenses, in order to be immunologically poly-competent one day, and moreover societally poly-comprehensible. To survive in the best possible way this phase of encounters, for the moment fraught with dangers and risks,

Conclusion written by Bruno SALGUES.

before being, in the next phase of the human, animal and viral mix, a beacon of universal understanding and resilience, we will need vigilance and prevention. With regard to micro-organisms, and also other types of threats (more human ones), everyone will have to become a hunter, a detector of the bizarre, the abnormal and the unexpected.

In this regard, clusters, a word that most of the world did not know, has become a household word with the advent of Covid-19. In fact, the outbreak has set up a problem with places, from French Air Base 110 to the University Hospital of Bordeaux, as well as the seafood market and live animals in Wuhan and the diverse habitats of bats. Other scientific words have passed into the language of the mainstream press, such as PCR tests, and non-scientific names, such as enzymes or antibodies. Various words emerged as keywords and markers for the texts that make up the book that is about to be concluded: affordance, otherness, altruism, common sense, good practice, trust, social distancing, neo-teleworkers, pangolin, wild reservoirs, severe acute respiratory syndrome and so on. Thus, each of these terms could constitute the starting point for reflections about the future work that the Covid-19 should generate.

The epidemic that compels us is a source of scientific methods and tools. It is also a source of innovations, some of them more or less far-fetched. In particular, in future discussion, we should ask ourselves questions about the future of the concept of emerging diseases in relation to the foundations of health action and policies as well as to the International Classification of Diseases, as the bible of the reality of the diseases that threaten us. What is the role of models and committees of scientists in helping to make political decisions? This is a controversy that could be addressed in our further discussion.

Lockdown has been a necessary point of public action, and the religious fact invites us to reflect between an imposed and voluntary lockdown. Tools have seen their use increase during the pandemic: teleworking, teleconsultations, chat rooms. As far as teleworking is concerned, it has become an injunction in European countries as part of the second lockdown.

Rituals, customs and habits have been disrupted by the epidemic, and some have emerged. Do we need to reinvent myths and rituals, either to be part of society or to find oneself? This is also a real question that needs to be debated. Similarly, the fact that respect for biodiversity and the fight against climate change have emerged as themes that are still necessary to integrate into society's actions, in addition to that of epidemics, and the fact that the threefold balance between the economy, ecology and the defense of public health is both necessary and complex to establish should be points that give rise to new analyses. In this regard, and this is just one example, we have seen – with great astonishment and some incomprehension – millions of masks arrive by plane from China. We have discovered that the same is true of the majority of painkillers that we use every day to soothe our teeth, our heads, our arthritis and our sciatica.

Finally, the limitation of human interaction through lockdown goes hand in hand with a surprising communicative expansion, a "communitagion", which can very well cohabit with conspiracy debates. Is this a necessary evil of the digital society or a weak signal of major societal change?

List of Authors

Jacques BARNOUIN
EPIA, INRAE
Clermont-Ferrand-Theix
France

Jean-Paul BOIS-MARGNAC
INRIA
Le Chesnay
France

Guy CAVEROT
Inter'NOV
Nantes
France

Emmanuel CHÉNÉ
IAE
University of Nantes
France

François DEMONGEOT
Consultant
Strasbourg
France

Éric FOGARASSY
CNRS
Strasbourg
France

Jean-Pierre GIRARDEAU
MEDIS, INRAE
Clermont-Ferrand-Theix
France

Emmanuel MIGNOT
Salon du Télétravail
Paris
France

Judith NICOGOSSIAN
Neurosciences UGA
Grenoble
France

Bruno SALGUES
Institut Mines-Télécom
Palaiseau
France

Henri SAMIER
ParisTech
France

Christian SCHOEN
Terra Firma
Boulogne Billancourt
France

Philippe TRONC
DigiLence
Paris
France

Index

G, H

I, K

L, M

N, O, P

Q, R

S, T

U, V

W, X, Z

Other titles from

iSTE

in

Health Engineering and Society

2022

ASSAILLY Jean-Pascal
Child Psychology: Developments in Knowledge and Theoretical Models
(Health and Patients Set – Volume 3)

CHAABANE Sondès, COUSEIN Etienne, WIESER Philippe
Healthcare Systems: Challenges and Opportunities

PAGANELLI Céline, CLAVIER Viviane
Information Practices and Knowledge in Health
(Health and Patients Set – Volume 5)

2021

BÉRANGER Jérôme
Societal Responsibility of Artificial Intelligence: Towards an Ethical and Eco-responsible AI
(Technological Prospects and Social Applications Set – Volume 4)

CORDELIER Benoit, GALIBERT Olivier
Digital Health Communications
(Technological Prospects and Social Applications Set – Volume 5)

NADOT Michel
Discipline of Nursing: Three-time Knowledge

2020

BARBET Jacques, FOUCQUIER Adrien, THOMAS Yves
Therapeutic Progress in Oncology: Towards a Revolution in Cancer Therapy?
(Health and Patients Set – Volume 2)

MORILLON Laurent, CLAVIER Viviane
Health Research Practices in a Digital Context
(Health Information Set – Volume 4)

PAILLIART Isabelle
New Territories in Health
(Health Information Set – Volume 3)

2019

CLAVIER Viviane, DE OLIVEIRA Jean-Philippe
Food and Health: Actor Strategies in Information and Communication
(Health Information Set – Volume 2)

PIZON Frank
Health Education and Prevention
(Health and Patients Set – Volume 1)

2018

HUARD Pierre
The Management of Chronic Diseases: Organizational Innovation and Efficiency

PAGANELLI Céline
Confidence and Legitimacy in Health Information and Communication (Health Information Set – Volume 1)

2017

PICARD Robert
Co-design in Living Labs for Healthcare and Independent Living: Concepts, Methods and Tools

2015

BÉRANGER Jérôme
Medical Information Systems Ethics

CPSIA information can be obtained
at www.ICGtesting.com
Printed in the USA
BVHW022032190323
660223BV00030B/13

9 781786 307262